The Simple Ketogenic Diet Cookbook For Beginners

by Martha Smith

Contents

What this book is all about

In this book you will discover 66 amazing recipes, which are very simple and delicious. They are designed to guide you every step of the way in order to prepare the best keto foods ever. All of these recipes are relaying on easy techniques and ingredients. The results are flavorful and satisfying. Each recipe includes the nutritional information and has up to 7 grams of net carbs. This is the best way to track your macronutrients and customize your diet to fit your unique needs. As well this Keto cookbook comes with a 2-week meal plan and the perfect diet food list, which is great for anyone starting out. The book will help you through your weight loss journey or dealing with other health issues such as: epilepsy, depression, Alzheimer's disease, Parkinson's disease and other related issues. It is time to start to renovate your life with this delightful Keto recipes. Let's go!

What is Ketosis?

In simple terms ketosis is a state of metabolism where the body relies on fat as a source of energy.

From a biological point of view, the human body is an extremely adaptable machine that adapts itself to all sorts of conditions. In our modern high-carb diet, the main source of energy is glucose. When glucose is available, the body is directed first to it because it is metabolized very fast. But when you are in ketosis, things are different - the body relies heavily on ketones instead of glucose. To understand how this process works, we need to be aware that some organs in the human body (especially the brain) need a certain amount of glucose to function. If our brain does not reach glucose, we will not be alive.

But that does not mean that you need to get your glucose through food - the body is able to get the right amount of glucose even during prolonged hunger or a period of minimal intake of carbohydrates.

There are two ways this can happen. The first is through the breakdown of muscle protein that is used as fuel for the brain and the liver. This is certainly not the ideal option because muscle mass is a metabolically active tissue that you do not want to lose. Fortunately, there is a second way to synthesize glucose: the ketone bodies.

Ketone bodies are water-soluble molecules produced in the liver by fatty acids. They cover some of the needs of the brain and other major glucose bodies (to prevent too much muscle breakdown).

How do we know we are in ketosis?

If you want to test your ketone levels, you can do it with blood meter, urine sticks and blood sticks. If you want also to test the levels of acetone in your breath, you can use a breathing analyzer.

Simply follow how your body responses, so you can see if you are in kethosis. Here are the main signs that will show you that you are definitely in ketosis.

Decreased starvation: Hormones, which regulate the appetite are repressed by ketones and help you feel fuller for a longer time.

Loosing weight: Keto diet helps to burn fat easily, and if you lose weight, you may be in ketosis.

Specific breath (keto breath): If you feel a metallic taste in your mouth it is because of the increased levels of ketones.

Most people to adapt to ketosis will need about 2-3weeks.The main problem is the brain - it has to adapt to the use of fuel ketones. Taking 3 to 5 grams of sodium and at least 1 gram of potassium per day will help a lot to make the ketogenic transition properly, keeping your brain health excellent!

Health benefits of the Keto diet

Following a keto diet has been shown to provide a significant health benefits such as better concentration, increase energy levels, better mental performance and also lower the inflammation.

As a bonus, kethosis suppresses the appetite and keeps the blood sugar stable. As a result, if you have not eaten for several hours, you do not feel exhausted and dizzy. In addition, the keto diet is extremely rich in beneficial fats and micronutrients (vitamins, minerals and antioxidants) and at the same time low in toxins.

Ketose is also useful in the treatment of a number of diseases. Research has shown that keto diet helps obese individuals with insulin resistance to improve insulin sensitivity and restore normal metabolism.

People in ketosis state have seen improvements in blood pressure, blood sugar and cholesterol levels. Keto diet is an extremely effective for many neurological diseases and conditions such as epilepsy, migraine, Parkinson's, Alzheimer's and even brain tumors.

Risks and disadvantages of the Keto Diet

We can not deny the benefits of the Keto diet, but it also carries certain risks.

Ketosis is best to be avoided in some rare diseases such as deficiency of pyruvate carboxylase, porphyria, and any other disorder of fat metabolism.

Therefore, it is not suitable for pregnant and lactating women, as well as for those who are trying to get pregnant. To conceive, you need to eat balanced. The same applies to nutrition during pregnancy - ketosis may be dangerous for both the mother and the fetus.

Other risks include loss of bone density, constipation (due to reduced fiber intake), thyroid problems, and vitamin C deficiency. If you have kidney problems, keto diets can cause complications. I also do not recommend this diet for children and adolescents, as there may be a slowdown in growth.

How to minimize the risks from the Keto diet

Fortunately, there are ways to reduce these risks to a minimum.

Certain foods and supplements (for example, the amino acids lysine and leucine) support ketosis, which allows the consumption of more protein and carbohydrates. The short-chain fatty acids contained in coconut oil also have a ketogenic effect because they signal the liver to produce more ketone bodies.

This gives you more flexibility and you know that diet is safer in the long run. Taking vitamin D will reduce the risk of bone loss.

The other solution is to take a more conservative approach - a cyclic keto diet. Cyclic keto diets usually alternate several keto days with one or two high carb days. This allows you to be more flexible and enjoy a more diverse diet. Cyclic keto diets are, in most cases, the better option because they retain the benefits but reduce the risk of ketosis.

What to Eat on a Keto Diet

You should base most of your nutrition on these foods:

Meat: All sausages, Turkey, Chicken, Offal, Pork, Bacon, Lamb, Beef andDuck.

Eggs: Organic eggs.

Fish and seafood: Snoek, Hake, Salmon, Calamari, Angel fish, Scallops, Trout, Tuna, Sardines, Yellowtall, Prawns, Scallops, Anchovies and Kob.

Fruits: Lemon, Raspberries, Lime, Coconut, Cranberries, Blackberries and Tomato.

Veggies: Kale, Cauliflower, Onions, Radishes Asparagus, Broccoli, Mushrooms, Cabbage, Aubergine, Brussel sprouts, Cucumber, Peppers, Artichokes, Pumpkin, Olives, Spinach, Green beans and Lettuce.

Fats: Coconut milk, Lard, Duck fat, Mayonnaise, Coconut oil, Animal fats, Butter, Macadamia, Avocado oil, Coconut cream, Heavy cream and Extra virgin olive oil.

Lunch & Deli Meats: Salami, Prosciutto, Ham, Chorizo, Speck, Pastarmi, Bacon, Pepperoncino, Soppressata and Pancetta.

Sauces and Condiments: Tomato sauce, Hot sauce, Mustard, Vinegar and Mayonnaise.

Dairy: Feta cheese, Parmesan cheese, Cream, Butter, Greek yogurt, Cream cheese, Blue cheese and other high fat cheese.

Nuts: Macadamia, Walnuts, Hazelnuts, Pecans, Brazils and Almonds.

Herbs and spices: Granules and Bouillon cubes.

Flour: Hazelnut flour, Almond flour, Coconut flour and other nut flours.

Seeds: Pumpkin seeds, Sunflower seeds, Chia seeds, Sesame seeds and Flax seeds.

Drinks: Tea, Sparkling water, Water and Coffee.

Sweet things: Stevia, Erythritol and Xylitol.

Canned food: Sardines, Olives, Sauerkraut, Crab, Pickles, Tuna, Salmon, Anchovies, Tomato (check the nutrition facts label).

What to Avoid on a Keto Diet

In short, any foods that are high in carbohydrates should be limited.

Here is a list of foods that need to be avoid on a Ketogenic Diet:

Sugars: Soft drinks, fruit juice, shakes, cake, ice cream and candies.
Starches: Starchy vegetables, soy, lentils, sago, tapioca, plantain, banana, and mesquite.
Dietary and low-fat products: Evaporated skim milk, low-fat yogurts, fat-free butter substitutes, and reduced fat cheese.
Grains and grain-like seeds: Rice, wheat, quinoa, oats, amaranth, barley, buckwheat, corn, and millet.
Sauces: They often contain sugar and unhealthy fats.
Flours: Wheat flour, cornmeal, arrowroot, cornstarch, cassava, dal, and fava beans.
Unhealthy Fats: Limit the intake of processed vegetable oils, sunflower oil and mayonnaise.
Processed vegetable oils and trans fats: Diglycerides, shortening, vegetable shortening, margarine, interesterified oils, corn oil, cottonseed oil, grapeseed oil, safflower oil, and soybean oil
Fruits: All fruits & dried fruits
Alcohol: Thanks to the carbohydrate content, many alcoholic beverages can throw you out of ketosis, especially beer and liqueurs.

Healthy Keto Snacks

In case you are hungry between main meals, here are some useful keto-approved snacks:

Keto cheese chips

Boiled eggs

Avocado

Pepperoni slices

Veggie sticks

Pickles

Milk shake with almond milk,
    cocoa powder and butter

Cherry tomatoes

Lettuce wraps

Bacon-wrapped keto foods

Cheese with olives

Whole-fat yoghurt with butter and cocoa powder

Strawberries with cream cheese

Keto kale chips

Iced coffee

Homemade popsicles

Bone broth

Seaweed snacks

Pork Rinds

Keto Diet Quick Hacks

Here are several advanced ketogenic diet hacks to get into and maintain ketosis.

Count your macros - preferably use an app on your phone to record everything you eat.

Stay hydrated - drink a lot of water, at least eight 8-ounce glasses

Do regular exercise - at least 30 minutes a day. Tracking it with a smart watch or fit bracelet is very easy and helpful.

Measure your Ketones (use the ways described above to determine your ketosis state)

Make a meal plan - or simply use the one provided in this book.

Reduce the stress - sleep more and cut stressful people and situations the same way you do with carbs.

Intermittent fasting can really boost your keto results.

Increase salt intake - make sure your electrolytes are on point when you are on the keto diet.

Sample Keto Food Plan for 2 weeks

To help you get started, here is a sample of a meal plan for two weeks:

Day 1
Breakfast: Delicious Keto Sandwiches
Lunch: Grilled shrimp skewers
Dinner: Cabbage Stir Fry with Beef

Day 2
Breakfast: No- Bake Coconut Balls
Lunch: Crispy Garlic Chicken Wings
Dinner: Baby Spinach Soup

Day 3
Breakfast: Healthy Kale Chips
Lunch: Cauliflower soup with bacon
Dinner: Creamy Chicken Breasts

Day 4
Breakfast: Strawberry Mousse
Lunch: Chicken Fillet with Tomato Sauce
Dinner: Beef salad

Day 5
Breakfast: Asparagus with Sauce "Hollandaise"
Lunch: Fresh Melanzane Salad
Dinner: Italian Sushi with Prosciutto di Parma

Day 6
Breakfast: Lemon Delights
Lunch: Roasted Turkey Breast with Garlic Sauce
Dinner: Stuffed Mushrooms with Bacon

Day 7
Breakfast: Broccoli Casserole with Cheddar
Lunch: Asian Pork Shoulder with Green Beans
Dinner: Stuffed Green Bell Peppers with Beef

Day 8
Breakfast: Deviled Eggs with Bacon and Green Onion
Lunch: Baby Ribs in the Oven
Dinner: Skillet Chicken Fillet with Zucchini

Day 9
Breakfast: Scrambled Eggs with Kale and Mozzarella
Lunch: Grandma's Meatballs with Yogurt Sauce
Dinner: Old Style Beef Soup

Day 10
Breakfast: Coconut Pudding
Lunch: Roasted Salmon with Steamed Spinach
Dinner: Easy Beef with Green Beans

Day 11
Breakfast: Egg Muffins with Bacon
Lunch: Avocado Salad with Shrimps
Dinner: Rich Pork Chops with Onion

Day 12
Breakfast: Stuffed Avocado with Egg
Lunch: Grilled Salmon with Kale Pesto
Dinner: Grilled Parmesan Pork Chops

Day 13
Breakfast: Creamy Stuffed Spinach Eggs
Lunch: Lemon's Broccoli with Almonds
Dinner: Marinated Chicken Skewers with Lemon

Day 14
Breakfast: Blackberry Coconut Treat
Lunch: Wrapped Chicken Bites with Bacon
Dinner: Cheddar Stuffed Zucchini

VEGETABLES & SIDE DISHES

1. Zucchini Salad with Tuna

Ready in about 15 min | Servings 4

Ingredients

- 1 cup tomatoes, cut into cubes
- 2 tablespoons lemon juice
- fresh mint leaves
- 1 can tuna in olive oil
- 3 zucchini
- salt and pepper to taste
- 3 tablespoons extra virgin olive oil
- 2 tablespoons avocado oil, for the dressing
- 1 cup mozzarella cheese, cut into cubes

Nutritional Information

300 Calories;
23g Fat;
5.6g Carbs;
1.8 Fiber;
17.1g Protein

Directions

Cut the zucchini into slices that are about 1/4 inch thick. Brush the zucchini with olive oil on each side. Sprinkle with salt and pepper.

Place the seasoned zucchini in large pan over medium heat. Grill until both sides turn a nice golden brown color.

Then put the zucchini on a plate. Add the tuna over the zucchini. Top with the mozzarella and tomatoes, cut into cubes.

To make the vinaigrette mix the lemon juice, salt and avocado oil in a small bowl.

Pour over the zucchini and garnish with fresh mint leaves.

2. Cauliflower Soup with Bacon

Ready in about 40 minutes | Servings 6

Ingredients

- 1 medium head cauliflower, cut into florets
- 2 tablespoons olive oil
- 3 cups vegetable broth
- 1 onion, chopped
- 2 cloves garlic, minced
- 1/3 cup heavy cream
- salt and pepper, to taste
- 1 teaspoon dried oregano
- 1 teaspoon thyme
- 2 tablespoons butter
- 1/3 cup cooked bacon

Nutritional Information

151 Calories;
13g Fat;
5.4g Carbs;
1.5g Fiber;
2.4g Protein

Directions

Preheat your oven to 400 F.

Place the cauliflower, garlic and onion in a large baking tray covered with baking paper.

Drizzle with olive oil. Season with salt and pepper.

Bake for 20 minutes in the preheated oven or until the cauliflower is fork-tender.

Place the cauliflower, onion and garlic in a soup pot. Add the butter, vegetable broth, oregano, thyme, salt and pepper.

Stir well and boil for 15 minutes. Let it cool for a few minutes.

Transfer the soup to a blender. Add the cream and blend until smooth. Work in batches.

Serve and garnish with the bacon.

3. Delicious Keto Sandwiches

Ingredients

- 6 leaves Romaine lettuce, rinsed
- 1/3 cup parmesan cheese, shredded
- 1 red onion, thinly sliced
- 1 large tomato, thinly sliced
- 1/3 cup mayonnaise
- 2 avocados, thinly sliced

Nutritional Information

175 Calories;
15.6g Fat;
7g Carbs;
4.8g Fiber;
3.9g Protein

Directions

Smear the mayonnaise on the lettuce leaves and place them on your kitchen counter.

Layer each leaf with the sliced onion, tomato and avocado.

Top with shredded parmesan cheese.

Fold the lettuce like small tacos and serve with your favorite dipping sauce.

4. Easy Green Baby Spinach Soup

Ingredients

- 5 cups spinach
- 2 small onions, finely chopped
- 2 medium-size carrots, finely chopped
- ½ cups coconut oil
- 2 garlic cloves, sliced
- 1 teaspoon pepper
- 1 teaspoon salt
- 12 cups water
- 1 cube vegetable broth
- ½ cup parmesan cheese, grated

Nutritional Information

173 Calories;
18g Fat;
3g Carbs;
1g Protein

Directions

Heat the coconut oil in a large pot.

Add the onions, carrot and garlic. Sautee for 3 minutes.

Add the water and the vegetable broth. Bring to a boil for 8 minutes.

Stir in the spinach and boil for another 12 minutes. Season with salt and pepper.

Transfer the soup to a blender and blend until smooth. Work in batches.

Serve hot and sprinkle with parmesan cheese.

5. Healthy Kale Chips

Ready in about 30 min | Servings 4

Ingredients

- 1 bunch kale
- 1 tablespoon olive oil
- 1 teaspoon salt
- 1 teaspoon pepper
- 1 teaspoon paprika

Nutritional Information

66 Calories;
3.6g Fat;
6.1g Carbs;
73g Protein

Directions

Preheat the oven to 350 F°.

Wash the kale and let it dry completely.

After the kale is dry place it in a large bowl. Season with the olive oil, salt, black and red pepper.

Arrange the kale leaves on one line in a large baking tray covered with baking paper.

Bake for 13-15 minutes in the preheated oven. The leaves must remain dark green.

When they are ready, let them cool for 2-3 minutes and enjoy.

6. Fresh Melanzane Salad

Ingredients

- 1 eggplant
- 2 medium tomatoes, diced
- 2 tablespoons olive oil
- 1 roasted red pepper, diced
- 1 red onion, chopped
- salt, to taste
- 2 tablespoons fresh parsley, chopped
- 1/3 cup feta cheese, diced

For the dressing
- 2 tablespoons olive oil
- 2 tablespoons lemon juice
- ½ teaspoon dried oregano
- ½ teaspoon dried basil

Nutritional Information

171 Calories;
13.4g Fat;
5.5g Carbs;
3.1g Protein;
4.2g Fiber

Directions

Cut the eggplant lengthwise and brush with olive oil. Season with salt.

Add the eggplant to a grill pan over medium heat, cook until the eggplant gets soft. Turning a few times.

In a small bowl mix the olive oil, lemon juice, dried oregano and dried basil. Set aside.

In a large bowl add the eggplant slices, diced tomatoes, roasted red pepper, chopped onion and fresh parsley.

Drizzle with the dressing and stir well.

Top with feta cheese and serve.

7. Italian Sushi with Prosciutto di Parma

Ready in about 15 minutes | Servings 4

Ingredients

- 12 slices of Prosciutto di Parma
- ½ cups cream cheese
- ½ medium avocado
- 1/3 cup cucumber
- 1 ½ tablespoons sesame seeds

Nutritional Information

402 Calories;
44g Fat;
4g Carbs;
2.1g Fiber;
13g Protein

Directions

Lay the prosciutto slices on a flat surface.

Cut the avocado and cucumber into thin short strips with the same length as the width of the prosciutto slices. Set aside.

Spread a thin layer of cream cheese on each slice of the prosciutto.

Place one avocado and one cucumber strip at one end of each prosciutto slice.

Roll up the prosciutto slices carefully and tightly.

Sprinkle with sesame seeds and serve.

8. Lemon's Broccoli with Almonds

Ready in about 20 min | Servings 2

Ingredients

- 2 cups fresh broccoli
- 2 tablespoons butter
- ½ cup peeled almonds
- 2 tablespoons freshly squeezed lemon juice
- 1 teaspoon salt
- 3 cloves garlic, pressed

Nutritional Information

141 Calories;
11.5g Fat;
3.9g Carbs;
4g Protein

Directions

Cut the broccoli into florets.

Bring a large pot with salted water to a boil. Add the broccoli and let them boil for 4 minutes.

Once ready drain them and let them cool for 5 minutes. Set aside.

Meanwhile, melt the butter in a saucepan and add the almonds. Cook for 2-3 minutes.

When the almonds are ready, add the boiled broccoli, freshly squeezed lemon juice, salt, and pressed garlic.

Stir gently for a couple of minutes and serve warm.

9. Stuffed Mushrooms with Bacon

Ingredients

- 4 tablespoons fresh chives, finely chopped
- 1 cup cream cheese
- salt and pepper to taste
- 1 cup bacon
- 1 ½ teaspoon paprika powder
- 14 large portobello mushrooms
- 3 tablespoons butter
- 2 tablespoons vegetable oil

Nutritional Information

176 Calories;
14.5g Fat;
6.7g Carbs;
3.3 Fiber;
7.5g Protein

Directions

Heat the vegetable oil in a large pan over medium heat. Fry the bacon until it gets crispy and reserve the bacon fat. Set aside.

Wipe the mushrooms and remove the stalks. Chop the mushroom stalks and sauté with butter in the bacon fat.

In a large bowl mix the fried bacon, sautéed stalks, paprika powder, cream cheese and chopped fresh chives. Season with salt and pepper to taste.

Spray a baking dish with nonstick cooking spray and preheat the oven to 350°F

Fill the mushroom caps with the mixture and arrange them in the baking dish.

Bake for 15 minutes or until golden brown.

10. Cheddar Stuffed Zucchini

Ready in about 50 min | Servings 4

Ingredients

- 4 zucchinis
- 1 cup tomato puree
- 2 cloves garlic, minced
- 1 small yellow onion, finely chopped
- 1 small red onion, finely chopped
- 1 large carrot, chopped
- ½ cup Cheddar Cheese, shredded
- 2 tablespoons canola oil
- 1 red pepper, diced
- ½ teaspoon oregano
- ½ teaspoon paprika
- fresh basil leaves, for garnish
- salt and pepper, to taste

Nutritional Information

204 Calories;
15.2g Fat;
6.3g Carbs;
2.8 Fiber;
6.3g Protein

Directions

Cut the zucchini into halves. Then using a spoon scoop out the flesh of the zucchini halves, but leave some at the bottom.

Dice the zucchini flesh into small pieces. Set aside.

Season the zucchini with salt and pepper.

Place the zucchini on a baking tray covered with baking sheet.

In a medium skillet preheat the canola oil.

Add the minced garlic, chopped carrot, diced zucchini flesh, diced red pepper, finely chopped yellow and red onion. Cook until soft.

Season with oregano, paprika, salt and pepper. Stir well.

Add the tomato sauce and cook for 7 minutes.

Fill the zucchini with the sauce and top with the shredded cheddar cheese.

Bake for 20 minutes or until golden brown in a preheat oven at 400 degrees F.

Serve and garnish with fresh basil leaves.

POULTRY

11. Bacon Wrapped Chicken Bites

Ready in about 20 min | Servings 6

Ingredients

- 2 lbs. boneless chicken breasts, cut into 1-inch chunks
- 1 teaspoon smoked paprika
- 1/3 cup grated parmesan cheese (optional)
- salt and pepper, to taste
- 8 pieces of bacon, cut into thirds
- fresh parsley, for garnish

Nutritional Information

333 Calories;
13.2g Fat;
3.8g Carbs;
0.8g Fiber;
47g Protein

Directions

Place the chicken chunks in a bowl. Season with salt, pepper and smoked paprika. Combine well.

Wrap the pieces of bacon over the chicken chunks and secure with a toothpick.

Preheat the oven to 350F.

Place the wrapped chicken bites in a large baking dish with parchment paper.

Bake for 15-20 minutes.

Serve hot and sprinkle with grated parmesan cheese.

12. Marinated Chicken Skewers with Lemon

Ready in about 50 min | Servings 6

Ingredients

- 2 lbs. boneless chicken breasts, cut into cubes
- 2 tablespoons olive oil
- 2 tablespoons soy sauce
- 2 tablespoons honey
- 1 teaspoon turmeric
- 1 teaspoon salt
- 1 teaspoon pepper
- 2 tablespoons with lemon juice
- 1 teaspoon paprika

Nutritional Information

253 Calories;
9.2g Fat;
3.7g Carbs;
0.5g Fiber;
32.6g Protein

Directions

Place the olive oil, soy sauce, honey, turmeric, salt, pepper, lemon juice and paprika in a large bowl. Whisk well.

Add the chicken cubes to the bowl. Stir well. Cover with plastic wrap.

Refrigerate for 20 minutes.

Soak the wooden skewers in water for 20 minutes.

Preheat a grill pan on medium heat.

Thread the chicken onto the skewers.

Grill for 4 to 5 minutes on each side or until is cooked.

Serve hot!

13. Skillet Chicken Fillet with Zucchini

Ready in about 15 min | Servings 6

Ingredients

- 6 chicken breasts
- 1/3 cup fresh oregano, chopped
- 3 medium zucchini, sliced into half moon shapes
- 3 garlic cloves, minced
- 1 medium onion, chopped
- 1 tablespoon fresh parsley, chopped
- 1 teaspoon salt
- 1 teaspoon pepper
- 3 tablespoons butter
- 2 tablespoons avocado oil
- 6 lemon slices, optional

Nutritional Information

253 Calories;
9.2g Fat;
4.8g Carbs;
0.5g Fiber;
32.6g Protein

Directions

Melt the butter in a medium skillet over medium heat.

Add the fresh oregano, minced garlic, chopped onion. Stir well.

Season the chicken breasts with salt and pepper. Add them to the skillet. Work in batches.

Cook 3-4 minutes per side or until the chicken breasts are ready. Set aside.

Add the sliced zucchini and avocado oil to the skillet. Sprinkle with salt and pepper and cook for 3 minutes.

Turn off the heat and add the parsley. Stir well.

Serve the chicken breasts with the zucchini and with fresh lemon slices on the side.

14. Creamy Chicken Breasts

Ready in about 20 min | Servings 4

Ingredients

- 2 large halved chicken breasts
- 1 teaspoon salt
- 1 teaspoon pepper
- 3 cloves garlic, chopped
- 2 tablespoons olive oil
- 1 cup heavy whipping cream
- ½ cup parmesan cheese
- ½ cup chicken broth
- 1 teaspoon dried basil

Nutritional Information

486 Calories;
32g Fat;
4.7g Carbs;
0.3g Fiber;
43.6g Protein

Directions

Season the chicken breasts with salt and pepper.

In a large skillet on medium heat, add the olive oil.

Cook the chicken for 5-6 minutes per side or until golden brown. Work in batches and set aside.

Add the chopped garlic, heavy whipped cream and chicken broth in the skillet. Stir well to combine.

Add the parmesan cheese and basil. Simmer for 4-5 minutes.

Return the chicken to the pan and simmer for another 1-2 minutes.

Serve warm and enjoy!

15. Crispy Garlic Chicken Wings

Ready in about 20 min | Servings 4

Ingredients

- 2 lbs. chicken wings
- 1 teaspoon Kosher salt
- 1 teaspoon pepper
- ½ teaspoon chili powder
- ½ teaspoon smoked paprika
- 1 teaspoon garlic powder
- ½ teaspoon cumin
- ½ teaspoon dried oregano
- 2 tablespoons olive oil
- 2 tablespoons soy sauce
- fresh cilantro, chopped (optional)

Nutritional Information

379 Calories;
16.4g Fat;
4.1g Carbs;
0.7g Fiber;
50g Protein

Directions

Pat dry the chicken wings with paper towels and place them in a large bowl. Add the olive oil and soy sauce. Toss gently to coat.

In a small bowl mix the seasonings. Sprinkle the seasoning mixture over the chicken wings and massage well.

Preheat the oven to 350 degrees F.

Bake the chicken wings for 40 minutes or until golden brown.

Serve with fresh cilantro.

16. Yummy Chicken Legs with Parmesan

Ready in about 1 hour | Servings 6

Ingredients

- 2 lbs. chicken legs
- 1/3 cup soy sauce
- 1/3 cup olive oil
- 2 teaspoons paprika
- 1 ½ teaspoon pepper
- 1 teaspoon salt
- 3-4 garlic cloves, minced
- 1/3 cup ketchup
- ½ cup grated parmesan (optional)

Nutritional Information

419 Calories;
22g Fat;
6.5g Carbs;
0.6g Fiber;
47.1g Protein

Directions

In a large bowl whisk the soy sauce, olive oil, paprika, pepper, salt, minced garlic and ketchup.

Add the chicken legs in a large zip-top bag and pour the marinade.

Refrigerate the chicken legs for at least 30 minutes.

Bake the chicken legs for 20 minutes in a preheated oven at 350°F.

Turn the chicken legs and bake for additional 10 minutes or until they get tender.

Serve immediately and sprinkle with parmesan.

17. Baked Spinach Chicken Breasts

Ready in about 40 min | Servings 4

Ingredients

- 2 chicken breast halves, boneless and skinless
- 2 tablespoons olive oil
- 1 teaspoon dried thyme
- 1 yellow onion, chopped
- 1 teaspoon pepper
- 2 garlic cloves, minced
- 1/3 cup chicken broth
- 1 ½ cup fresh spinach, washed and chopped
- 1 teaspoon Kosher salt
- 1 teaspoon dried rosemary

Nutritional Information

416 Calories;
21g Fat;
6g Carbs;
2.2g Fiber;
47.6g Protein

Directions

Spray a baking pan with cooking spray and heat the oven to 350 F.

Place the spinach in the baking pan. Sprinkle with salt and pepper.

Then lightly grease the chicken breasts with olive oil. Season with salt, pepper, thyme and rosemary.

Place the chicken breasts over the spinach.

Add the chopped onion, minced garlic cloves and the chicken broth.

Cover with foil and bake for 15 minutes.

Remove the foil and bake for another 15 minutes or until the chicken is deep golden brown.

Let it rest for 5 minutes and serve.

18. Chicken Fillet with Tomato Sauce

Ready in about 25 min | Servings 4

Ingredients

- 3 tablespoons olive oil
- 1 teaspoon salt
- 1 teaspoon pepper
- 3 gloves garlic, minced
- 2 tablespoons butter
- 1 red onion, chopped
- 3 cups plump tomatoes, diced
- ½ teaspoon dried basil
- 2 chicken breast halves, boneless and skinless
- ½ teaspoon oregano
- 3 tablespoons tomato paste
- 1/3 cup fresh parsley (optional)

Nutritional Information

448 Calories;
27.2g Fat;
5.6g Carbs;
2.1g Fiber;
42.6g Protein

Directions

In a large skillet preheat the olive oil.

Season the chicken breasts with salt, pepper, basil and oregano.

Cook 5-6 minutes per side or until golden brown. Work in batches and set aside.

In the same skillet add the butter, minced garlic and chopped red onion.

Cook 1-2 minutes and then add the diced tomatoes and tomato paste. Simmer for 5-6 minutes.

Place the chicken breasts back to the skillet and cook for another 2-3 minutes with the tomato sauce.

Place the chicken breasts in the tomato sauce and mix well.

Serve warm and sprinkle with fresh parsley.

19. Turkey Mayo Salad

Ingredients

- 2 medium cups roasted turkey breast, chopped
- salt and pepper, to taste
- 1 tablespoon lemon juice
- 1 cup mayonnaise
- 1 stalk celery, chopped
- 1 tablespoon Dijon mustard
- 2 tablespoons greek yogurt
- 1 teaspoon fresh basil
- 1 teaspoon fresh parsley
- 1 tablespoon olive oil

Nutritional Information

492 Calories;
29g Fat;
3.7g Carbs;
1.2g Fiber;
46g Protein

Directions

In a large bowl mix the chopped roasted turkey, celery, basil and parsley.

In a medium bowl mix the mayonnaise, lemon juice, Dijon mustard, greek yogurt, olive oil, salt and pepper. Stir.

Add the mayo mixture to the turkey mixture. Combine well.

Place in the refrigerator for 40 minutes or more.

Serve on a bed of lettuce or with avocado slices (optional).

20. Roasted Turkey Breast with Garlic sauce

Ready in about 1h | Servings 3

Ingredients

- 2 teaspoons Kosher salt
- 1 teaspoon pepper
- 1 lbs. skinless turkey breast
- 3 garlic cloves, crushed
- 3 tablespoons melted butter
- 2 teaspoons rosemary
- 2 tablespoon light soy sauce
- 1 teaspoon thyme

For the garlic sauce
- 1 tablespoon melted butter
- 1/2 cup chicken broth
- 5 garlic cloves, chopped
- 1/2 tablespoon almond flour
- ½ cup heavy cream
- 1 teaspoon fresh parsley, chopped
- salt and pepper to taste

Nutritional Information

375 Calories;
18.6g Fat;
3.1g Carbs;
0.5g Fiber;
47g Protein

Directions

In a small bowl combine the kosher salt, pepper, garlic cloves, melted butter, rosemary, light soy sauce and thyme. Mix well.

Rub the mixture into the turkey breast. Place the turkey breast in a large roasting pan in a preheated oven to 355°F.

Bake for 50 minutes or until is cooked. Set aside.

In a saucepan add the melted butter and the almond flour. Stir constantly for 2-3 minutes.

Add the chicken broth, chopped garlic, parsley, salt and pepper to taste.

Cook until it gets thick and then add the heavy cream. Mix well.

Serve the turkey warm with the garlic sauce.

PORK

21. Asian Pork Shoulder with Green Beans

Ingredients

- 1/2 lbs. pork shoulder
- 3 garlic cloves, sliced
- 1 ½ tablespoon tamari
- 2 tablespoons sesame oil
- 1 ½ tablespoon rice vinegar
- 1 cup green beans
- ½ teaspoon pepper
- ½ teaspoon salt
- 2 scallions, sliced
- 2 teaspoons sesame seeds

Nutritional Information

424 Calories;
30g Fat;
7g Carbs;
2.5g Fiber;
24.9g Protein

Directions

Cut the pork shoulder into strips and season with salt and pepper.

In a large pan add the sesame oil and fry the pork for 3-4 minutes.

Add the garlic cloves, sliced scallions and green beans. Stir in the tamari and rice vinegar. Stir well. Season with salt and pepper.

Cook until the pork turns golden brown.

Sprinkle with sesame seeds and serve.

22. Baby Ribs in the Oven

Ingredients

- 1 rack of baby back ribs
- ½ cup ketchup
- 2 tablespoons olive oil
- 1/2 teaspoon onion powder
- 1 teaspoon cayenne pepper
- ½ teaspoon garlic powder
- 1 teaspoon salt
- ½ cup BBQ sauce (optional)

Nutritional Information

480 Calories;
32g Fat;
5.4g Carbs;
0.4g Fiber;
38.9g Protein

Directions

Place the ribs in a large baking tray.

In a medium bowl combine the ketchup, onion powder, cayenne pepper, olive oil, garlic powder and salt. Mix well.

Rub the mixture all over the ribs on both sides.

Cover the baking tray with foil and bake for 1 hour in a preheated oven at 380°F.

Leave to rest for 10 minutes and serve.

23. Bone-in Pork Chops with Brussels Sprouts

Ready in about 30 min | Servings 4

Ingredients

- 2 bone-in pork chops
- 1 teaspoon salt
- 1 teaspoon pepper
- 2 tablespoons vegetable oil
- 2 cloves garlic, minced
- 1 teaspoon dried rosemary
- 2 cups Brussels sprouts, trimmed and halved
- 2 tablespoons mustard

Nutritional Information

480 Calories;
16.2g Fat;
6.9g Carbs;
2.9g Fiber;
29.6g Protein

Directions

Preheat the oven to 300F.

In a large bowl combine the Brussel sprouts with the salt, pepper, dried rosemary, minced garlic, honey, mustard and one tablespoon vegetable oil.

Spread on the Brussel sprouts on a cooking sheet in a large baking tray.

Bake for 20 minutes or until golden brown. Set aside.

Season the pork chops with salt and pepper.

In a large skillet heat the remaining vegetable oil.

Add the pork chops and cook for 4-5 minutes per side or until browned.

Serve the pork chops with the Brussel sprouts on the side.

24. Grandma's Meatballs with Yogurt Sauce

Ingredients

- 1 lbs. pork mince
- ½ teaspoon salt
- ½ teaspoon pepper
- 1/3 cup parmesan cheese, grated
- 1 medium egg
- 2 tablespoons olive oil
- 1/3 cup parsley, finely chopped
- 1/3 cup heavy cream

For the Yoghurt sauce
- ½ cup Greek-style yogurt
- 1 tablespoon olive oil
- 2 garlic cloves, minced
- ½ teaspoon salt
- 1 tablespoon fresh dill, chopped

Nutritional Information

421 Calories;
31g Fat;
4.1g Carbs;
0.5g Fiber;
28.6g Protein

Directions

Preheat the oven to 350F.

In a large bowl mix the pork mince, salt, pepper, parmesan cheese, egg, finely chopped parsley and heavy cream. Mix well.

Form into 15 balls.

Place the meatballs in a large baking tray covered with baking paper.

Bake for 6-7 minutes per side or until golden brown. Set aside.

In a small bowl mix the greek yogurt, olive oil, minced garlic, salt and chopped dill. Stir well.

Serve the meatballs with the yogurt sauce on the side.

25. Grilled Parmesan Pork Chops

Ingredients

- 2 pork chops
- 1 teaspoon oregano
- 1 teaspoon onion powder
- 1/3 teaspoon chili powder
- 1 ½ tablespoon avocado oil
- 1/3 cup parmesan cheese, grated
- 1 teaspoon garlic powder
- 1 ½ tablespoons dried parsley
- ½ teaspoon dried thyme
- ½ teaspoon paprika
- salt and pepper, to taste
- 3 tablespoons fresh cilantro
- 1/2 tablespoon sesame seeds

Nutritional Information

526 Calories;
33g Fat;
5.8g Carbs;
1.5g Fiber;
46g Protein

Directions

Season the pork chops with salt and pepper.

In a large bowl mix the avocado oil, parmesan, oregano, onion powder, chili powder, garlic powder, dried parsley, thyme and paprika.

Soak the pork chops in the bowl for 15 minutes and refrigerate.

Preheat a grill pan to medium-high.

Grill until golden brown, around 4-5 minutes per side.

Serve with fresh cilantro and sprinkle with sesame seeds.

26. Pork Lion with Cabbage

Ingredients

- 1 lbs. pork lion, boneless and cut into strips
- 4 tablespoons olive oil
- 1 small onion, chopped
- 3 cups green cabbage, shredded
- salt and pepper, to taste
- ½ teaspoon coriander
- 1/2 cup chicken broth
- 1 tablespoon apple cider vinegar

Nutritional Information

380 Calories;
23.2g Fat;
7.2g Carbs;
2.5g Fiber;
33g Protein

Directions

Season the pork lion strips with salt, pepper and coriander.

In a large skillet on medium heat add two tablespoons of olive oil. Cook the pork lion strips for 3-4 minutes per side or until cooked. Set aside.

In a medium skillet add the chopped onion, shredded cabbage, two tablespoons olive oil, chicken broth, apple cider vinegar, salt and pepper to taste. Stir to combine.

Cook for 15 minutes or until the liquid has evaporated.

Serve immediately with the pork lion strips on the side.

27. Rich Pork Chops with Onion

Ready in about 35 min | Servings 6

Ingredients

- 6 pork chops
- 1 cup chicken broth
- 1/3 cup heavy whipping cream
- 1/3 teaspoon salt
- 2 yellow onions, sliced into thin pieces
- 1/3 teaspoon black pepper

Nutritional Information

415 Calories;
22.6g Fat;
0.7g Carbs;
0g Fiber;
49g Protein

Directions

In a large skillet, add the onions and cook for 15 minutes or until the onions are soft. Stir constantly. Season with salt and pepper and set aside.

Sprinkle the pork chops with salt and pepper.

In a pan over medium heat, add the chops and fry for 4-5 minutes per side or until they are ready.

Remove to a large dish and tent with foil.

Add the chicken broth to the pan and stir. Then add the heavy whipping cream until the mixture gets thick.

Return the onions to the pan and mix well.

Serve the pork chops with onion mixture.

28. Sausage Skillet with Zucchini

Ingredients

- 6 sausages links
- 1 large zucchini, sliced
- 2 garlic cloves, minced
- 1 medium onion, chopped
- 1/3 cup olive oil
- salt and pepper, to taste
- 1 teaspoon dried oregano
- 1 teaspoon dried basil
- 1 cup cherry tomatoes, cut into halves

Nutritional Information

253 Calories;
19.2g Fat;
6.1g Carbs;
1.2g Fiber;
14.7g Protein

Directions

In a large skillet over medium heat, place the sausages and fry until browned. Set aside.

Add the olive oil, minced garlic and chopped onion to the skillet. Cook for 2-3 minutes.

Add in the sliced zucchini and stir well. Cook for 6-7 minutes.

Season with salt, pepper, basil and oregano.

Add the cherry tomatoes and cook until soft.

Place the sausages back to the skillet and cook for another 2-3 minutes until hot.

Serve immediately.

29. Traditional Pork Soup

Ready in about 30 min | Servings 6

Ingredients

- 2 bone-in pork chops, cut into small cubes
- 1 teaspoon salt
- 1 teaspoon pepper
- 2 small carrots, chopped
- 1 green bell pepper, chopped
- 1 large onion, diced
- 2 cups chicken broth
- 3 cups water
- 1 bay leaf
- 1 teaspoon cumin
- 1 teaspoon chili powder
- 2 cloves garlic, minced
- 1 tablespoon butter

Nutritional Information

280 Calories;
13.5g Fat;
6g Carbs;
1.3g Fiber;
31.7g Protein

Directions

In a large saucepan, add the butter, minced garlic, pork chops, chopped carrots, green bel pepper and onion.

Sautee for 6-7 minutes.

Then transfer them to a large stock pot and stir in the chicken broth and water.

Season with salt, pepper, bay leaf, cumin and chili powder.

Boil for 20 minutes or until pork is tender.

Serve hot.

30. Pork Steaks with Spicy Asparagus

Ingredients

- 2 medium pork steaks
- 1 teaspoon Kosher salt
- 1 teaspoon pepper
- 2 tablespoons vegetable oil
- 2 cups fresh asparagus,
- 1 jalapeno, seeded and minced
- 2 cloves garlic, minced
- 3 tablespoons butter

Nutritional Information

403 Calories;
31.8g Fat;
4g Carbs;
1.6g Fiber;
26g Protein

Directions

In a medium skillet put the butter and the minced garlic. Stir well.

Add the fresh asparagus and jalapeno pepper. Cook around 2-3 minutes or until the asparagus is tender. Set aside.

Heat the vegetable oil in a large pan and fry the pork steaks around 5-6 minutes per side or until they are ready.

Season with salt and pepper.

Serve the pork steaks along with the spicy asparagus.

BEEF

31. Stuffed Green Bell Peppers with Beef

Ingredients

- 2 large green bell peppers, washed
- 1 small yellow onion, chopped
- 2 tablespoons olive oil
- 2 garlic cloves, minced
- salt and pepper, to taste
- 3/4 lbs. ground beef
- 1 teaspoon dried oregano
- ¼ cup cheddar cheese, shredded
- 1 teaspoon paprika
- ½ teaspoon cumin
- ¼ cup tomato sauce
- 2 tablespoons green onion, chopped (for garnish)

Nutritional Information

387 Calories;
31g Fat;
6.6g Carbs;
3.2g Fiber;
13.9g Protein

Directions

Cut off the tops of the peppers and remove the seeds.

Season the peppers on the inside with salt and pepper. Drizzle with olive oil and set aside.

Heat the olive oil in a large pan.

Add the minced garlic and chopped yellow onion. Fry until soft.

Then add the beef, dried oregano, paprika and cumin. Cook for 6 minutes.

Stir in the tomato sauce and simmer for 7-8 minutes.

Stuff the peppers with the mixture and add top with the shredded cheddar cheese.

Bake for 20 minutes (or until the cheese has melted) in your oven at 360F.

Garnish with green onion.

32. Quick Beef with Broccoli

Ingredients

- 2 tablespoons butter
- 5 cups broccoli florets
- 1 lbs. ground beef
- salt and pepper, to taste
- 1 yellow onion, chopped
- 2 garlic cloves, minced
- ½ teaspoon dried thyme
- 1 teaspoon dried basil
- 2 tablespoons sesame oil

Nutritional Information

402 Calories;
27.8g Fat;
4g Carbs;
2.1g Fiber;
32.3g Protein

Directions

In a large skillet melt the butter. Add the broccoli florets, onion and garlic. Fry for 6-7 minutes.

Season with salt, pepper and basil. Set aside.

In another skillet heat the sesame oil.

Add the ground beef and season with salt, pepper and thyme. Cook until it reaches your desired level of doneness.

Serve the beef warm with the broccoli on the side.

33. Old Style Beef Soup

Ready in about 45 min | Servings 6

Ingredients

- 3 small beef steaks
- 2 small carrots, diced
- 1 large onion, diced
- 1 large red pepper, diced
- 2 tablespoons olive oil
- 1 large zucchini, diced
- 2 cloves garlic, minced
- 1 teaspoon paprika
- ½ cup tomatoes, diced
- salt and pepper, to taste
- 5 cups beef broth
- ½ teaspoon dried thyme
- ½ teaspoon dried rosemary
- fresh parsley, for garnish

Nutritional Information

246 Calories;
11.4g Fat;
4.7g Carbs;
2g Fiber;
26g Protein

Directions

Cut the beef steaks into small chunks. Season with salt and pepper.

In a large saucepan heat 1 tablespoon of olive oil and add the beef chunks. Cook until brown and set aside.

In a large pot heat 1 tablespoon of olive oil and add the minced garlic, diced onion, carrots, red pepper, zucchini.

Sauté for 3-4 minutes and stir in the beef broth and tomatoes. Stir well.

Season with salt, pepper, paprika, thyme and rosemary.

Boil for 30 minutes.

Serve warm and garnish with parsley.

34. Beef Flank with Tomato- Pepper Sauce

Ready in about 30 min | Servings 3

Ingredients

- 1 lbs. flank steak
- 2 red peppers, sliced
- 2 cloves garlic, minced
- 1 teaspoon paprika
- ½ teaspoon cumin
- 2 tablespoons olive oil
- 3 large tomatoes, chopped
- ½ teaspoon cilantro
- 1 red onion, chopped
- salt and pepper, to taste
- 1 jalapeno pepper, chopped optional

Nutritional Information

338 Calories;
17.4g Fat;
6.2g Carbs;
3g Fiber;
34.8g Protein

Directions

Cut the flank steak into ¼- inch thick pieces. Set aside.

In a large skillet add the olive oil, minced garlic and chopped red onion. Fry for 2-3 minutes.

Add the sliced red peppers and cook for 4-5 minutes.

Place the flank steak pieces in the skillet.

Season with salt, pepper, paprika, cumin and cilantro. Cook until brown.

Then add the chopped tomatoes and cook for 15 minutes.

Serve immediately and garnish with chopped jalapeno pepper (optional).

35. Flavorful Beef Zoodles

Ingredients

- 3/4 lbs. beef flank steak, sliced into 1-inch strips
- 2 medium zucchini, spiralized
- 2 medium carrots, spiralized
- 2 tablespoons coconut oil
- 1/3 teaspoon salt
- 1/3 teaspoon pepper
- 1 teaspoon red pepper flakes
- ¼ cup fresh cilantro, chopped

For the sauce
- 2 tablespoons soy sauce
- 2 cloves garlic, minced
- 2 tablespoons lemon juice

Nutritional Information

296 Calories;
16.9g Fat;
5.3g Carbs;
1.8g Fiber;
26.3g Protein

Directions

In a small bowl prepare the sauce by mixing the minced garlic, soy sauce and lemon juice. Set aside.

In a large skillet add the coconut oil and sliced flank steak.

Cook until the beef is brown and then add the spiralized carrots and zucchini.

Season with salt, pepper and red pepper flakes.

Stir in the prepared sauce and cook for 3-4 minutes.

Sprinkle with fresh cilantro and serve.

36. Cabbage Stir Fry with Beef

Ready in about 30 min | Servings 5

Ingredients

- 2 garlic cloves, minced
- 2 scallions, chopped
- 1 tablespoon white wine vinegar
- 2 ½ cups green cabbage, shredded
- 1 medium yellow onion, chopped
- 1 lbs. ground beef
- 1 teaspoon dried rosemary
- ½ teaspoon dried basil
- salt and pepper, to taste
- 3 tablespoons butter

Nutritional Information

493 Calories;
40g Fat;
6.5g Carbs;
2.8g Fiber;
19.2g Protein

Directions

Melt two tablespoons of butter in a large frying pan. Add the shredded cabbage and cook until soft.

Season with salt, pepper and add the vinegar. Stir well and cook for 3-4 minutes. Set aside.

Heat the rest of the butter in another frying pan. Add the minced garlic and chopped yellow onion. Cook for 2-3 minutes and add the ground beef.

Season with salt, pepper, dried basil and rosemary.

Fry until the meat is thoroughly cooked.

Lower the heat and add the chopped scallions and fried cabbage.

Stir until everything is hot and serve.

37. Delicious Beef Chuck with Mushroom Sauce

Ready in about 1 hour | Servings 5

Ingredients

- 1 large onion, diced
- 3 tablespoons olive oil
- 2 cloves garlic, minced
- 1 ½ cup beef broth
- salt and pepper, to taste
- ½ teaspoon dried thyme
- 2 cups mushrooms, cut into ½ inch pieces
- 2 lbs. beef chuck, thinly sliced
- ½ teaspoon tarragon
- 2 tablespoons fresh dill, finely chopped
- 1 cup heavy cream

Nutritional Information

457 Calories;
28g Fat;
7g Carbs;
1.8g Fiber;
40.3g Protein

Directions

Place a large skillet over high heat.

Add the olive oil, minced garlic, mushrooms and diced onion. Sauté for 3-4 minutes.

Season with salt, pepper, dried thyme and tarragon. Cook until golden brown.

Pour in the beef broth and simmer for 50 minutes.

Remove from heat and add the heavy cream. Stir well.

Serve immediately and garnish with fresh dill.

38. Easy Beef with Green Beans

Ready in about 20 min | Servings 2

Ingredients

- 1/2 lbs. ground beef
- 1 cup fresh green beans, rinsed and trimmed
- 1 medium yellow onion, chopped
- salt and pepper, to taste
- 2 cloves garlic, minced
- 2 tablespoons canola oil
- 1 teaspoon ginger, minced
- 1 teaspoon sesame seeds

Nutritional Information

440 Calories;
39g Fat;
5.9g Carbs;
2.8g Fiber;
15g Protein

Directions

In a large skillet add the canola oil, minced garlic and chopped onion. Fry for 2-3 minutes.

Then add the ground beef and cook until brown.

Stir in the green beans and minced ginger. Mix well and cook for 4-5 minutes.

Season with salt and pepper, to taste.

Sprinkle with sesame seeds and serve.

39. Beef Burgers with Prosciutto Crudo

Ready in about 20 min | Servings 6

Ingredients

- 1 lbs. ground beef
- 1 tablespoon onion powder
- 2 tablespoons fresh oregano, finely chopped
- ½ teaspoon salt
- ½ teaspoon pepper
- 1 tablespoon olive oil

For the topping
- 3 tablespoons Dijon mustard
- 1cup lettuce, shredded
- 1 tomato, sliced
- 6 medium slices fresh mozzarella
- 6 medium slices prosciutto crudo

Directions

In a medium bowl mix the ground beef, onion powder, chopped oregano, salt and pepper. Mix well.

Shape the burgers with wet hands and rub gently the meat with the olive oil.

Preheat the grill on medium heat. Grill the burgers for 4 minutes per side or until ready.

Serve on lettuce leaves and top with the mozzarella, Dijon mustard tomato and prosciutto crudo.

Serve and enjoy!

Nutritional Information

421 Calories;
30.3g Fat;
7.2g Carbs;
0.8g Fiber;
30.3g Protein

40. Beef Lime Salad

Ingredients

- 1 cup cherry tomatoes, cut into halves
- 3 cups mixed baby spinach
- ½ lbs. ribeye steaks
- 1 scallion, diced
- ½ cup blue cheese, crumbled
- 1 tablespoon olive oil
- 1/3 cup black olives, sliced
- lime wedges, for serving

For the dressing

- 3 tablespoons lime juice
- ½ teaspoon salt
- 2 tablespoons olive oil
- 1/3 teaspoon cumin
- 1 teaspoon Dijon mustard

Directions

- Heat a medium pan over high heat.
- Add the olive oil and ribeye steaks. Fry them 1-2 minutes per side.
- Cut the ribeye steaks into thin slices and set aside.
- In a small bowl add the lime juice, salt, olive oil, cumin and Dijon mustard. Combine well.
- In a large bowl mix the cherry tomatoes, mixed baby greens, diced scallion, sliced black olives, crumbled blue cheese and sliced ribeye steaks.
- Drizzle with the dressing and stir.
- Garnish with the lime wedges and serve.

Nutritional Information

433 Calories;
31.2g Fat;
5.8g Carbs;
1.3g Fiber;
33.5g Protein

FISH & SEAFOOD

41. Roasted Salmon with Steamed Spinach

Ingredients

- 1 lbs. salmon fillet
- 4 cups spinach
- 4 cloves garlic
- 1/2 teaspoon pepper
- 1/2 teaspoon salt
- 1 teaspoon butter
- 5-6 lemon slices

Nutritional Information

210 Calories;
9.2g Fat;
7.1g Carbs;
1g Fiber;
24.8g Protein

Directions

Clean the salmon and cut it into thick strips.

Add salt and pepper to the salmon.

Bake in a frying pan on both sides for a few minutes (or until it gets pink).

Clean and rinse the spinach.

In a saucepan add the butter, garlic and the rinsed spinach. Sauté for 6-7 minutes until soft.

On a plate, put the spinach, and on top of it place the fillets of salmon.

Garnish with lemon slices.

42. Avocado Salad with Shrimp

Ingredients

- 2 tomatoes, sliced into cubes
- 2 medium avocados, cut into large pieces
- 3 tablespoons red onion, diced
- ½ large lettuce, chopped
- 2 lbs. shrimp, peeled and deveined

For the Lime Vinaigrette Dressing
- 2 cloves garlic, minced
- 1 ½ teaspoon Dijon mustard
- 1/3 cup extra virgin olive oil
- salt and pepper to taste
- 1/3 cup lime juice

Nutritional Information

377 Calories;
17.6g Fat;
7g Carbs;
8g Fiber;
43.5g Protein

Directions

Add the peeled and deveined shrimp and 2 quarts of water to a cooking pot and print to a boil, lower the heat and let them simmer for 1-2 minutes until the shrimp is pink. Set aside and let them cool.

Next add the chopped lettuce in a large bowl. Then add the avocado, tomatoes, shrimp and red onion.

In a small bowl whisk together the Dijon mustard, garlic, olive oil and lime juice. Mix well.

Pour the lime vinaigrette dressing over the salad and serve.

43. Baked Codfish with Lemon

Ingredients

- 4 fillets code fish
- 1 teaspoon salt
- 1 teaspoon pepper
- 2 tablespoons olive oil
- 2 teaspoons dried basil
- 2 tablespoons melted butter
- 1 teaspoon dried thyme
- 1/3 teaspoon onion powder
- 2 lemons, juiced
- lemon wedges, for garnish

Nutritional Information

308 Calories;
23.6g Fat;
3.9g Carbs;
0.5g Fiber;
21.2g Protein

Directions

Preheat the oven to 400F.

In a medium bowl combine the lemon juice, onion powder, olive oil, dried basil and thyme. Stir well.

Season the fillets with salt and pepper.

Top each fillet into the mixture.

Lightly grease medium baking dish with the melted butter.

Bake the cod fish fillets for 15- 20 minutes.

Serve with fresh lemon wedges.

44. Baked Salmon with Tomatoes

Ingredients

- 1 lbs. salmon, in pieces
- 2 tomatoes, chopped
- 1/3 cup olive oil
- 1 tablespoon thyme
- salt, to taste
- 1/3 cup fresh dill, finely chopped
- 1/3 cup green olives, chopped
- 1 teaspoon ground black pepper

Nutritional Information

421 Calories;
32.8g Fat;
4.9g Carbs;
1.5g Fiber;
26.5g Protein

Directions

Preheat the oven to 400°F.

Finely cut the tomatoes and olives. Place them in a small bowl and add a little bit of olive oil, thyme, ground black pepper and salt. Mix well.

Place the salmon pieces in a baking dish. Pour the olive oil over the fish.

Add the tomatoes to the baking dish with the salmon.

Bake in the oven for 20 minutes or until the fish is done.

Garnish with fresh dill.

45. Fresh Green Salad with Tuna

Ready in about 10 min | Servings 4

Ingredients

- 1 can tuna, drained
- 2 cucumbers, peeled and chopped
- 1 green onion, sliced
- 1/2 baby lettuce, leaves torn
- 2 tablespoons extra-virgin olive oil
- 1/3 cup fresh parsley, chopped
- 20 medium Kalamata olives, pitted
- 8 cherry tomatoes, halved
- 2 tablespoons balsamic vinaigrette dressing
- salt and pepper, to taste

Directions

In a large bowl combine the chopped cucumbers, baby lettuce, baby tomatoes, Kalamata olives and fresh parsley. Mix well.

Add the tuna. Drizzle with extra-virgin olive oil and balsamic vinaigrette.

Season with salt and pepper to taste.

Garnish with green onion and serve.

Nutritional Information

127 Calories;
5.6g Fat;
6.9g Carbs;
4.2g Fiber;
11g Protein

46. Garlic Shrimp with Zucchini

Ingredients

- 3 zucchini, cut into thick strips
- 4 cloves garlic, minced
- 3 tablespoons fresh parsley, chopped
- 1 lbs. medium shrimp, peeled and deveined
- 3 tablespoons butter
- 1 teaspoon pepper
- Red pepper flakes, to taste
- Kosher salt, to taste
- 1 tablespoon vegetable oil

Nutritional Information

213 Calories;
10.9g Fat;
6.3g Carbs;
0.6g Fiber;
21.7g Protein

Directions

In a large pan over medium heat, melt the butter.

Then add the shrimp, red pepper flakes and garlic. Cook for 3-4 minutes or until the shrimp are cooked. Set aside.

In the same pan add the vegetable oil and zucchini stripes. Season with pepper and Kosher salt.

Saute for 3 minutes and add the cooked shrimp back to the pan. Mix well and cook for 2 minutes more.

Serve immediately and garnish with fresh parsley.

47. Grilled Salmon with Kale Pesto

Ready in about 30 min | Servings 4

Ingredients

- 2 lbs. salmon fillets
- 3 tablespoons olive oil
- ¾ teaspoon sea salt
- lemon pepper to taste

Kale Pesto
- 1 oz. walnuts
- ½ teaspoon black pepper
- 2 tablespoons olive oil
- 2 garlic cloves
- 1 cup kale, chopped
- 2 tablespoons lemon juice
- 1 teaspoon salt

Nutritional Information

508 Calories;
29.8g Fat;
3.4g Carbs;
1.1g Fiber;
54.5g Protein

Directions

Put the chopped kale, garlic, olive oil, walnuts and lemon juice in a blender. Blend until smooth. Season with salt and pepper. Set aside.

Season the salmon fillets with the sea salt and lemon pepper. Brush with olive oil.

Preheat a grill pan on medium heat.

Place the salmon fillets on preheated grill pan for 5 to 7 minutes per side or until the fish is done.

Serve the salmon fillets with the kale pesto.

48. Grilled Sardines with Herbs

Ingredients

- 8 fresh sardines, cleaned and trimmed
- ½ lemon
- 1 ½ tablespoon fresh rosemary, chopped
- 1 ½ tablespoon fresh parsley, chopped
- 2 teaspoons salt
- 2 teaspoons black pepper
- 2 tablespoons olive oil

Nutritional Information

167 Calories;
19.2g Fat;
3.3g Carbs;
1g Fiber;
12.3g Protein

Directions

Preheat the grill to high.

In a bowl prepare the juice by mixing lemon, olive oil, rosemary, parsley, salt and pepper.

Grease the sardines inside and outside with the mixture.

Grill the sardines for 3 minutes on each side.

Serve with coriander.

49. Grilled Teriyaki Shrimp Skewers

Ready in about 1 hour | Servings 6

Ingredients

- 2 lbs. medium shrimp, peeled and deveined
- 3 cloves garlic, minced
- ½ teaspoon salt
- ½ teaspoon pepper
- 12 bamboo skewers
- 1 tablespoon honey
- 2 tablespoons lemon juice
- 1/3 cup olive oil
- ½ teaspoon lime zest
- lemon wedges for serving
- 1/2 tablespoon cilantro, chopped
- ½ cup teriyaki sauce

Nutritional Information

251 Calories;
13.5g Fat;
7g Carbs;
0.2g Fiber;
22.3g Protein

Directions

Soak the bamboo skewers in water for 20 minutes.

In a large bowl combine the minced garlic, honey, lemon juice, olive oil, lime zest and teriyaki sauce.

Season with salt, pepper and cilantro. Mix well.

Add the shrimp to the bowl and marinade for 20 minutes in the refrigerator.

Preheat the grill over medium heat.

Thread the shrimp onto skewers, about 3 per stick.

Place the shrimp skewers on the grill. Cook for 2-3 minutes per side.

Serve with lemon wedges.

50. Pan-Fried Monkfish Medallions with Lemon Sauce

Ready in about 20min | Servings 2

Ingredients

- 1 ½ lbs. monkfish, cut into medallions
- salt and pepper, to taste
- 2 tablespoons olive oil
- lemon wedges, for serving

For the lemon sauce
- 3 tablespoons butter, melted
- ½ lemon, juiced
- salt and pepper, to taste
- 1 tablespoon Dijon mustard

Nutritional Information

328 Calories;
17.5g Fat;
3.9g Carbs;
0.5g Fiber;
37.3g Protein

Directions

Season the monkfish with salt and pepper.

Place a frying pan over a medium heat and add the olive oil.

Add the monkfish medallions to the pan and cook on both sides until golden brown. Set aside.

In a small bowl mix the melted butter, lemon juice, Dijon mustard, salt and pepper. Stir well.

Serve the monkfish medallions with the lemon wedges and drizzle with the lemon sauce.

EGGS & DAIRY

51. Asparagus with Sauce "Hollandaise"

Ingredients

- 1lbs. green asparagus
- 3 tablespoons butter
- salt and pepper to taste

For the sauce
- 3 egg yolks
- 2 tablespoons water
- 2 tablespoons olive oil
- juice of 1/2 lemon
- salt and red pepper to taste

Nutritional Information

236 Calories;
21.8g Fat;
6.9g Carbs;
2.5g Fiber;
5.6g Protein

Directions

In a bowl whisk the yolks and add cold water. Stir well.

Melt the butter in a saucepan and pour a thin stream of yolks. Constantly stir.

Season with salt, red pepper and lemon juice.

Clean and cut the asparagus 2-3 inches from the base.

Grill the asparagus for 1-2 minutes on each side.

Serve with the sauce.

52. Melanzane with Mozzarella

Ingredients

- 8 oz eggplant
- 2 cloves garlic, minced
- salt and pepper, to taste
- 2 tablespoons tomato sauce
- 1/3 cup mozzarella cheese
- 1 teaspoon dried oregano
- 2 tablespoons fresh parsley, chopped
- 6 black olives, diced
- 2 tablespoons olive oil

Nutritional Information

218 Calories;
13.8g Fat;
7g Carbs;
5.5g Fiber;
11g Protein

Directions

Rinse the eggplant and pat dry with a towel.

Cut the eggplant in a half. Scoop the meat of the eggplant and then dice. Reserve the scooped eggplant.

Drizzle the eggplant with olive oil and season with salt and pepper.

Preheat the oven to 400F.

In a medium skillet add the olive oil and minced garlic. Fry for 3-4 minutes.

Add the reserved eggplant meat, dried oregano, salt and pepper to taste.

Stir in the tomato sauce, diced olives and chopped parsley. Cook for 6-7 minutes.

Stuff the eggplant with the cooked mixture and place mozzarella cheese on top.

Bake for 25 minutes in the preheated oven and serve hot.

53. Egg Muffins with Bacon

Ready in about 20 min | Servings 6

Ingredients

- 6 large eggs
- ½ cup cooked bacon, chopped
- ½ cup cheddar cheese, shredded
- salt and pepper, to taste
- ½ teaspoon dried basil
- ½ teaspoon dried oregano
- chives for garnish (optional)

Nutritional Information

156 Calories;
12.8g Fat;
3.9g Carbs;
0.5g Fiber;
10g Protein

Directions

Preheat the oven to 350F.

In a medium bowl whisk together the eggs, salt, pepper, dried basil and dried oregano. Mix well.

Add the chopped bacon and shredded cheddar cheese. Stir.

Fill each muffin cup with the egg mixture.

Bake for 15 minutes or until the eggs are set.

Garnish with chives and serve.

54. Broccoli Casserole with Cheddar

Ready in about 20 min | Servings 4

Ingredients

- 16 cups broccoli florets
- ½ teaspoon salt
- ½ teaspoon pepper
- 1 cup sour cream
- ½ cup heavy cream
- 2 tablespoons butter
- 3 garlic cloves, minced
- ½ cup cheddar cheese, shredded
- 1 onion, chopped
- ½ teaspoon tarragon

Nutritional Information

357 Calories;
29.2g Fat;
7g Carbs;
3.5g Fiber;
15g Protein

Directions

In a large stockpot of boiling water add the broccoli florets. Boil for 3-4 minutes; drain and set aside.

In a medium saucepan melt the butter.

Add the minced garlic and chopped onion. Cook for 3-4 minutes.

Whisk in the sour cream and heavy cream. Combine well.

Season with salt, pepper, tarragon and add the shredded cheese.

In a casserole dish add the broccoli and pour the cream sauce.

Bake in a preheated oven to 400 F for 30 minutes.

Serve immediately and enjoy!

55. Coleslaw with Eggs

Ingredients

- 3 cups cabbage, shredded
- 2 large eggs, boiled
- 1 ½ tablespoon Dijon Mustard
- ½ cup mayonnaise
- ½ teaspoon salt
- ½ teaspoon pepper
- 2 tablespoons fresh parsley, chopped
- 1 teaspoon poppy seeds
- 1 tablespoon white vinegar

Nutritional Information

167 Calories;
12.8g Fat;
6.8g Carbs;
2.5g Fiber;
6.4g Protein

Directions

In a small bowl mix the Dijon mustard, mayonnaise and white vinegar. Set aside.

Peel the eggs and chop them.

In a large bowl mix the shredded cabbage, chopped parsley and chopped eggs.

Stir in the prepared dressing and combine well.

Season with salt, pepper, poppy seeds.

Put in the refrigerator for 1 hour before serving.

56. Creamy Stuffed Spinach Eggs

Ingredients

- 10 eggs
- 1 teaspoon lime juice
- 1 cup spinach
- 1 teaspoon salt
- 1 teaspoon red pepper
- 1 teaspoon pepper
- 1 teaspoon olive oil

Nutritional Information

137 Calories;
10.8g Fat;
1.7g Carbs;
0.1g Fiber;
9.4g Protein

Directions

Put the eggs in a saucepan and cover with water. Boil for 14 minutes.

After the eggs are boiled, drain the hot water. Add cold water to the eggs and leave them to cool for 1-2 minutes.

Peel and cut the eggs into halves. Separate the yolks.

Clean and cut the spinach.

Sauté the spinach in a saucepan with olive oil and add the separated yolks. Mix well.

Add the salt, pepper and red pepper to the mixture.

Stir until the mixture gets thick and smooth. Then, leave it to cool for a couple of minutes.

Put the egg whites cut-side-up on a serving dish. With a spoon, take from the mixture and stuff each egg. Sprinkle with lime juice.

57. Scrambled Eggs with Kale and Mozzarella

Ready in about 15 min | Servings 3

Ingredients

- 2 cups kale leaves, coarsely chopped
- 10 large eggs
- 2 teaspoons olive oil
- 1 small onion, finely chopped
- 1 teaspoon salt
- 1 teaspoon pepper
- 2 cloves garlic, minced
- 1 teaspoon oregano
- ½ cup mozzarella cheese, grated

Nutritional Information

260 Calories;
18.2g Fat;
6.6g Carbs;
1.5g Fiber;
16.4g Protein

Directions

In a saucepan add the olive oil, finely chopped onion, minced garlic and kale leaves.

Cook for 2-3 minutes and then add the eggs. Stir well.

Add the grated mozzarella cheese to the saucepan and stir until the eggs are ready.

Season with salt, pepper and oregano.

Serve immediately and enjoy!

58. Stuffed Avocado with Egg

Ingredients

- 2 large avocados
- 4 small eggs
- 1 teaspoon salt
- 1 teaspoon pepper
- ½ teaspoon red pepper flakes
- fresh basil (optional)

Nutritional Information

222 Calories;
18.3g Fat;
6.9g Carbs;
7g Fiber;
7.4g Protein

Directions

Preheat the oven to 400 F.

Cut the avocado into halves and remove the pit.

Season the avocado halves with salt, pepper and red pepper flakes.

Crack one egg in each avocado.

Bake for 15 minutes in a small baking dish with parchment paper.

Serve immediately with fresh basil (optional).

59. Stuffed Zucchini Boats with Pepperoni and Mozzarella

Ingredients

- 4 zucchini
- ½ cup mozzarella, grated
- 2 tablespoons olive oil
- 4 tablespoons Parmesan cheese
- ½ cup fresh cilantro, chopped
- 8 pepperoni slices
- 1 teaspoon salt
- 1 teaspoon pepper
- Fresh basil, for garnish

Nutritional Information

160 Calories;
10.5g Fat;
7g Carbs;
2.4g Fiber;
9.5g Protein

Directions

Slice the zucchini in half length-wise and remove the seeds with a spoon.

Season the zucchini with salt and pepper and drizzle with olive oil.

Fill the hollowed space in the zucchini with the grated mozzarella, parmesan cheese and fresh cilantro. On the top of each zucchini place 2 pepperoni.

Preheat the oven to 400°F.

On a large baking sheet, place the zucchini and bake for 15 minutes or until the zucchini get tender.

Serve and garnish with fresh basil.

60. Deviled Eggs with Bacon and Green Onion

Ready in about 30 min | Servings 8

Ingredients

- 8 large hard-boiled eggs, peeled
- 2 cloves garlic, minced
- 1 teaspoon Dijon mustard
- 2 tablespoons mayonnaise
- ½ teaspoon salt
- ½ teaspoon pepper
- 1/3 cup cheddar cheese, grated
- 5 slices bacon, cooked and crumbled
- ½ teaspoon rosemary
- 2 tablespoons green onion, finely chopped

Nutritional Information

157 Calories;
12.9g Fat;
1.5g Carbs;
0.2g Fiber;
8.7g Protein

Directions

Slice the hard boiled eggs in half. Scoop out the yolks and place them in a small bowl.

Add the minced garlic, Dijon mustard and mayonnaise. Stir well.

Season with salt, pepper and rosemary.

Stir in the grated cheddar cheese, finely chopped green onion and cooked bacon. Mix until well combined.

Put the mixture in a pastry bag. Snip off one corner and fill in each of the egg halves.

Sprinkle with additional chopped green onion or bacon crumbles. (optional)

DESSERTS

61. Avocado Ice Pops with Lime

Ready in about 5 min | Servings 10

Ingredients

- ¼ cup lime juice
- 3 avocados, ripe, peeled and stone re-moved
- 2 tablespoons honey
- 1 ½ cup coconut milk
- 3 tablespoons water, if seems thick

Nutritional Information

197 Calories;
17.4g Fat;
7g Carbs;
4.9g Fiber;
2.7g Protein

Directions

Put all of the above ingredients in a blender and mix until it reaches a smooth consistency.

If the mixture seems very thick add a little water.

Pour the mixture into popsicle molds.

Freeze for 5 hours or up to overnight.

Enjoy!

62. Blackberry Coconut Treat

Ready in about 45 min | Servings 8

Ingredients

- 1 cup fresh blackberries
- 1/2 teaspoon vanilla extract
- 1/2 cup coconut oil, softened
- 2 tablespoons water
- 1 teaspoon vanilla liquid stevia
- ½ tablespoon lemon juice
- Pinch of salt
- 1/2 cup coconut butter, softened

Nutritional Information

238 Calories;
25.4g Fat;
4.2g Carbs;
0.6g Fiber;
1g Protein

Directions

Put all the ingredients in a blender. Blend until smooth and thick.

Line an 8 capacity muffin pan with silicone cupcake liners.

Pour the mixture into each cup, about the half way.

Refrigerate 3-4 hours or freeze for 40 minutes. Enjoy!

63. Coconut Pudding

Ready in about 20 min | Servings 6

Ingredients

- 1/3 teaspoon salt
- 3 teaspoon Coconut liquid stevia
- 4 teaspoon gelatin
- 32 oz coconut milk unsweetened, canned
- 2 teaspoon vanilla extract

Optional toppings
- fresh berries
- unsweet coconut flakes

Nutritional Information

300 Calories;
32.4g Fat;
5.1g Carbs;
0g Fiber;
1g Protein

Directions

In a sauce pan put the coconut milk over medium heat. Stir constantly until it comes to a boil.

Reduce heat to simmer and add the gelatin. Stir well until the mixture gets thick.

Remove from the heat and stir in the vanilla extract, salt and coconut liquid stevia.

Pour into 6 medium jars.

Leave to cool 40 minutes then refrigerate for 3-4 hours.

Serve with fresh berries or unsweet coconut flakes.

64. No-Bake Coconut Balls

Ingredients

- 3 tablespoons xylitol
- 1 teaspoon vanilla
- 1 teaspoon salt
- 1 ½ cups organic unsweetened shredded coconut
- 3 tablespoons coconut oil

Nutritional Information

177 Calories;
15g Fat;
6.9g Carbs;
1g Fiber;
0.7g Protein

Directions

In a blender combine all the ingredients until the mixture sticks together.

Remove the mixture from the blender and with hands form small balls.

Decorate the balls with some extra shredded coconut.

Leave them in the refrigerator for 20-25 minutes.

65. Strawberry Mousse

Ingredients

- 2 cups coconut cream
- 1 cup fresh strawberries
- 1 ½ teaspoon vanilla powder
- fresh strawberries (for decoration)

Nutritional Information

412 Calories;
41.5g Fat;
7.4g Carbs;
3.4g Fiber;
4.7g Protein

Directions

Add the coconut cream and fresh strawberries in a blender.

Blend until a smooth consistency is reached.

Add the vanilla powder. Blend again.

Pour into glasses and place in the refrigerator for 30 minutes.

Decorate with fresh strawberries and serve.

66. Lemon Delights

Ingredients

- 4 large eggs
- 1 ½ cups lemon juice
- 1/2 cup butter, melted
- 1 1/2 cups almond flour
- Pinch of salt
- 1 ½ cup Swerve
- 2 tablespoons coconut oil, grease baking pan
- 8 lemon slices

Nutritional Information

136 Calories;
13.5g Fat;
2g Carbs;
0.1g Fiber;
1.7g Protein

Directions

Preheat the oven to 400 °F and rub an 8x8 inch pan with the coconut oil.

Mix 1 cup almond flour, ½ cup melted butter, pinch of salt and 1 cup Swerve until well combined.

Place the dough into the prepared form and bake until light brown. Set aside.

In a bowl mix ½ cup almond flour, 4 eggs, ½ cup Swerve, pinch of salt and the lemon juice. Mix well.

Pour the mixture onto the cooled crust and bake around 20 minutes or until is done.

Let it cool at room temperature and place in the refrigerator for a few hours.

Serve with fresh lemon slices.

Skylar's Great Adventure

The True Story of a Brave Fresh Pond Owlet

By John Harrison & Kim Nagy

Written by Kim Nagy

2

DEDICATION

Skylar's Great Adventure is dedicated to the next generation of owl watchers.

Mari Hylan, Oscar Kinsman, Sammy Kinsman, Zayah Asher Perlmutter, Caleb Jack Perlmutter, Mila Sage Perlmutter, Zachary Michael Kaplan, Cameron James Kaplan, Hannah Baron Silva, Ty Minogue, Kaelyn Minogue, Spencer Minogue, Nell Madigan Minogue,Hazel Leslie, Lydia Leslie, Justin Williamson, Zinnia Lili Roehl-Gordon, Lamine Gordon, Madeline Rhunette Aandahl, Spencer David Aandahl, Bernadine DeMatteo, Annetta DeMatteo, Maggie Carey, Hugh Carey III, Annie Carey, Sofie Proulx, Sage Proulx, Sky Proulx, Shayne Proulx, Cannon Proulx, Patrick O'Neill, Emma O'Neill, Addison Hale, Isobel Hale, Brooks Camorali, Nathan Robert Gaskill, Pierce Edward Antonsen, Quinlan Grace Hagan, Shea Alice Hagan, Ryann Rose Hagan, Antonio Strate, Jack Sorrentino, Max Sorrentino, Mary Abigail McElwreath, Caroline Marguerite McElwreath, Evelyn Rose Riggs, Corinne Grace Riggs, Norah Lynn Riggs, Hailey Rene Riggs, Rhea Coogan, Della Coogan, Emme Adams, Kylie Buckley, Campbell DeCoste, Cameron Demers, Quin Dijkstra, Maddie Douglas, Tim Eager, Finn Earner, Johanna Filliettaz, Ben Frazier, Isaiah Iliev-Rovnak, Julia Marino, Lilly Moon, Dill Parsons, Tyler Ridley, Alyssa Roy, Ned Spaulding, Chloey Succi, Adrian Vogel, Crystal Rose Cecchin, Charlotte Baker, Madeline DiGiorgio, Amelia DiGiorgio, Jocelyn Gesner, Ian Gesner, Evelyn Lamer, Owen Lamer and Ivan Lakits.

The G.H. Owls lived in a tall pine tree in a small city forest. G.H. stands for Great Horned, for that is the type of owl they were.

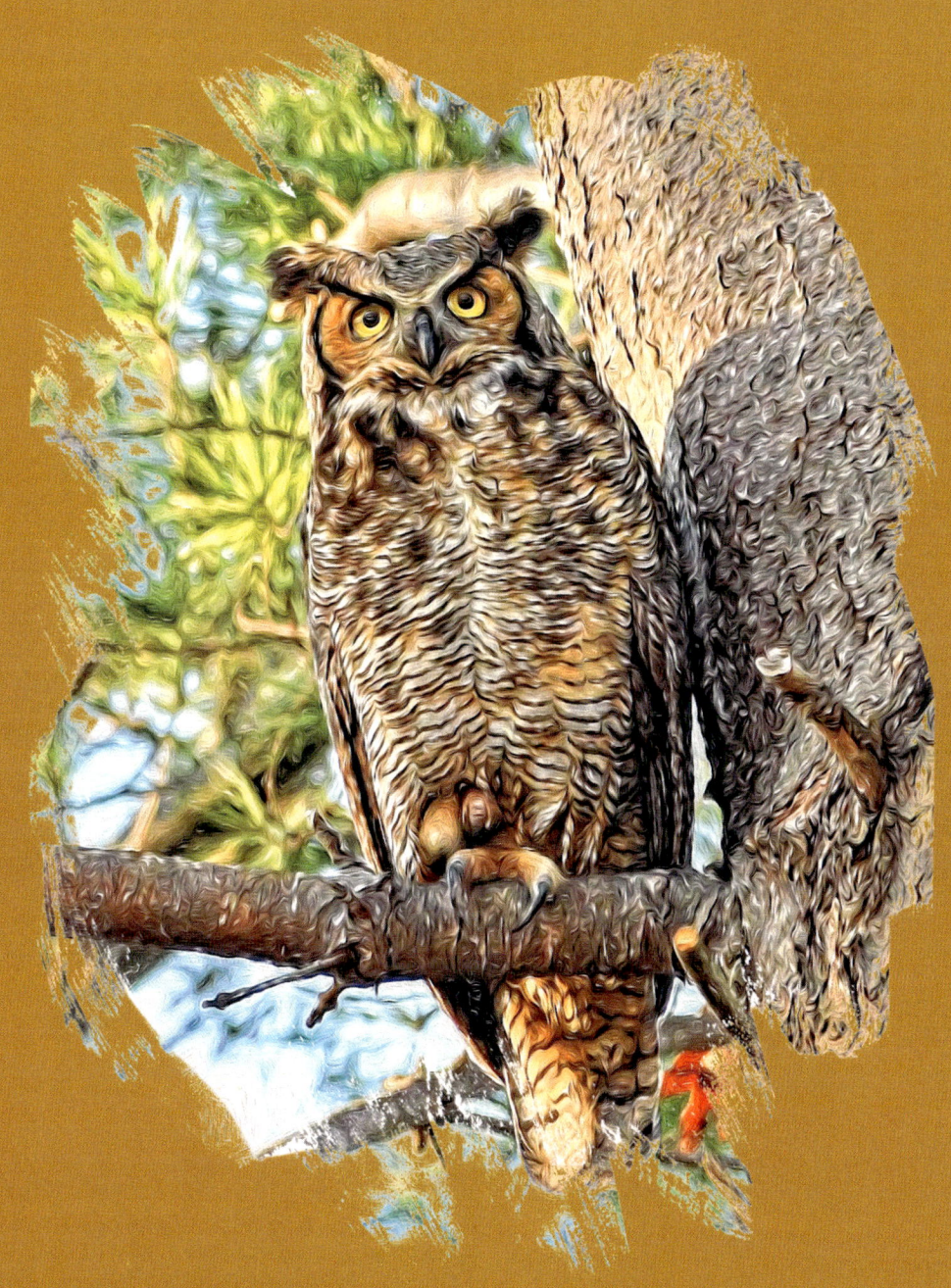

The small city forest surrounded a lake called Fresh Pond, in Cambridge, Massachusetts.

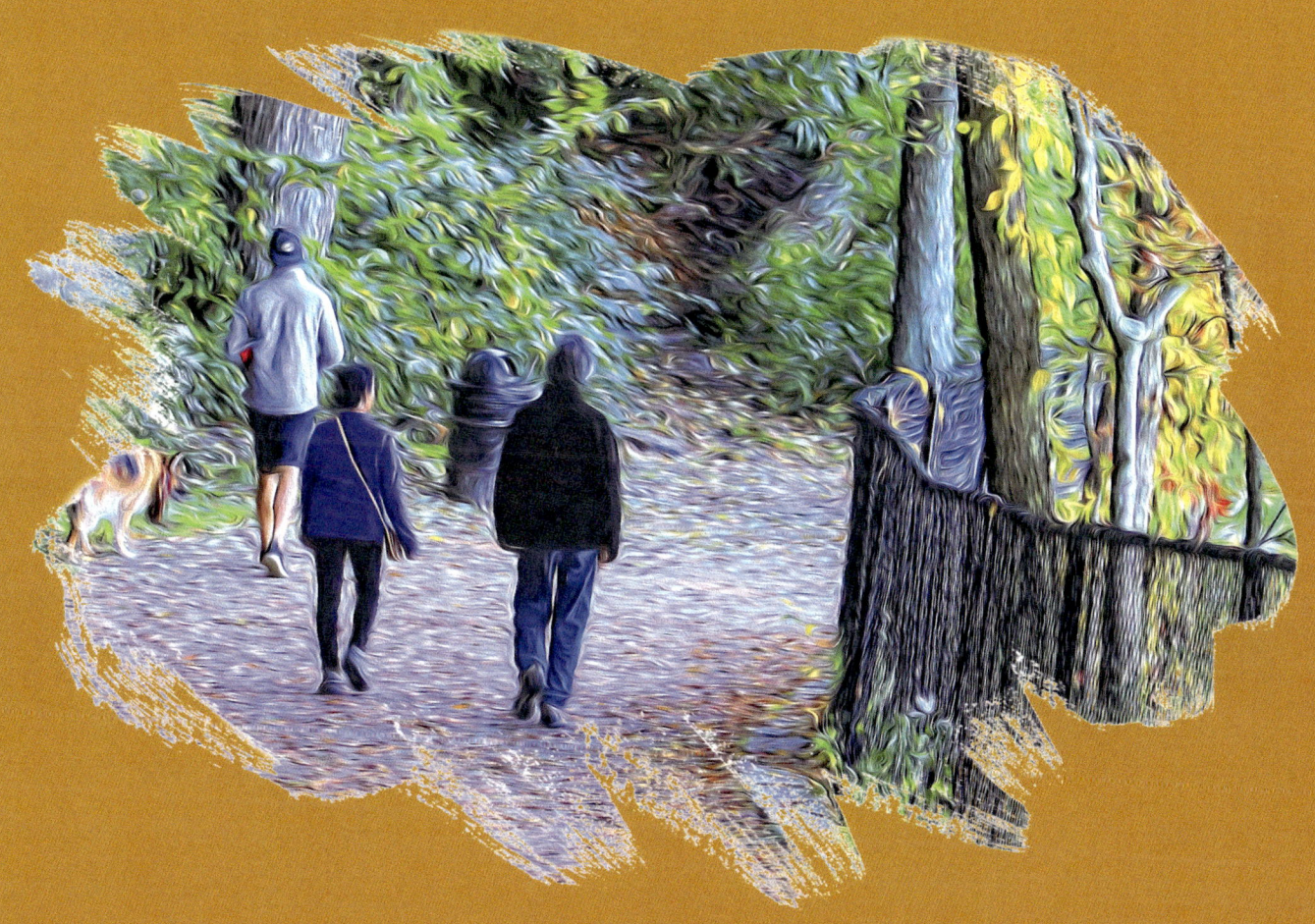

The owls were especially happy, because it was late winter and they were expecting two owl babies. Owl babies are called owlets.

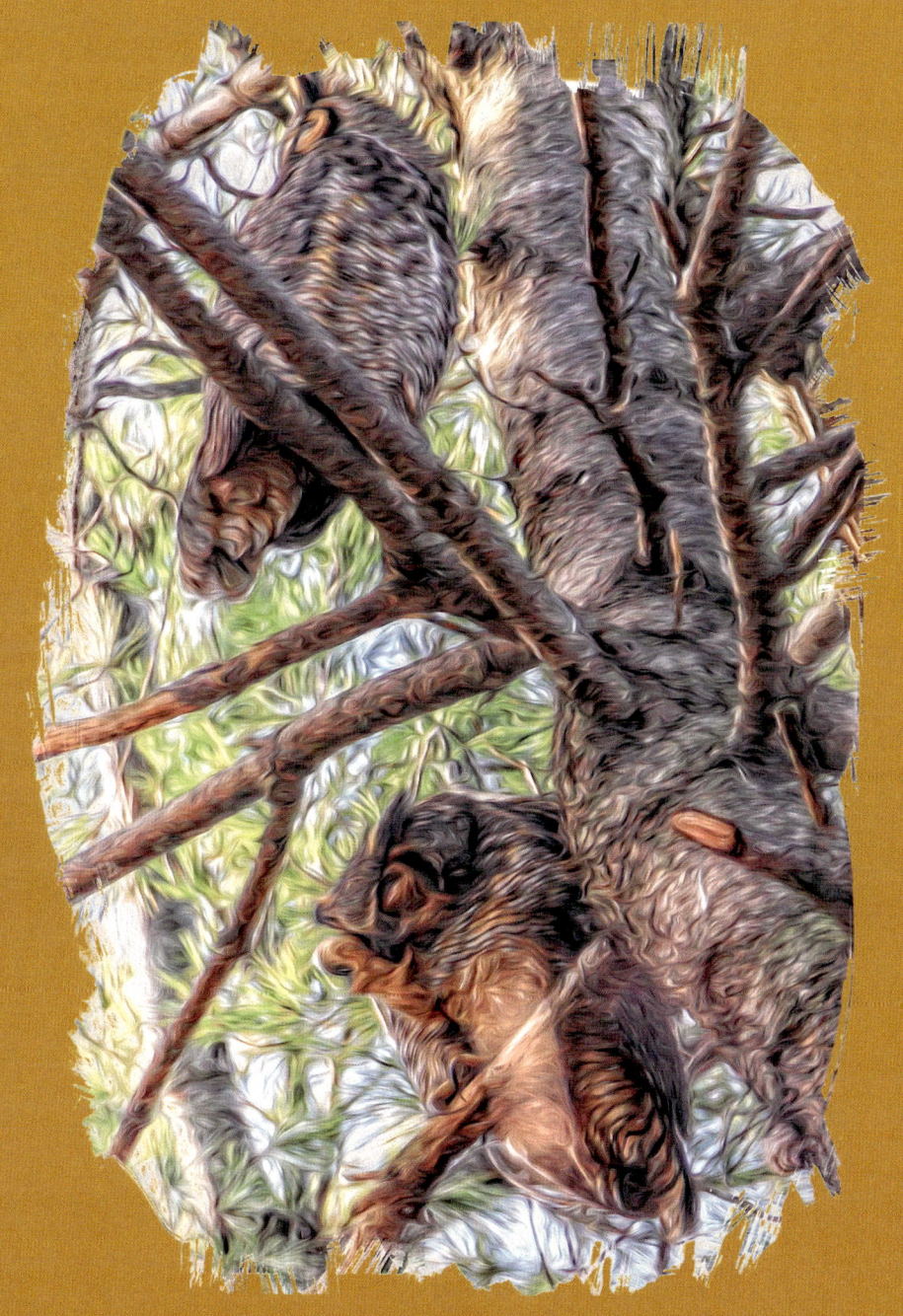

9

Mother Owl sat patiently on her eggs for over a month, to protect them and keep them warm. One day in late March, they finally hatched. Two new owls were born!

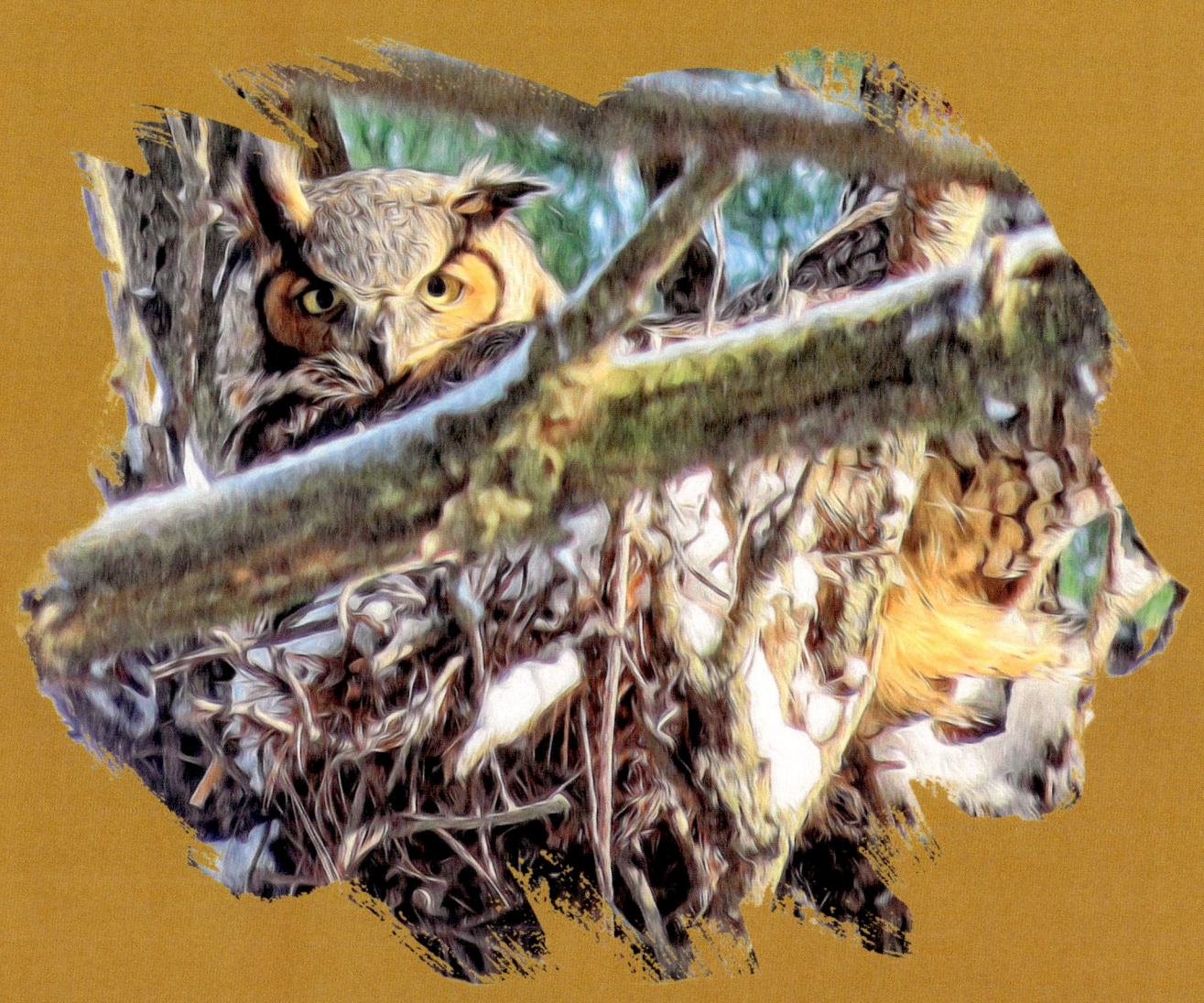

Father Owl worked hard to feed his family, and he regularly brought food back to the nest for Mother Owl and their two owlets. They needed lots of food because they were always hungry. Owls eat small mammals, including rats and mice.

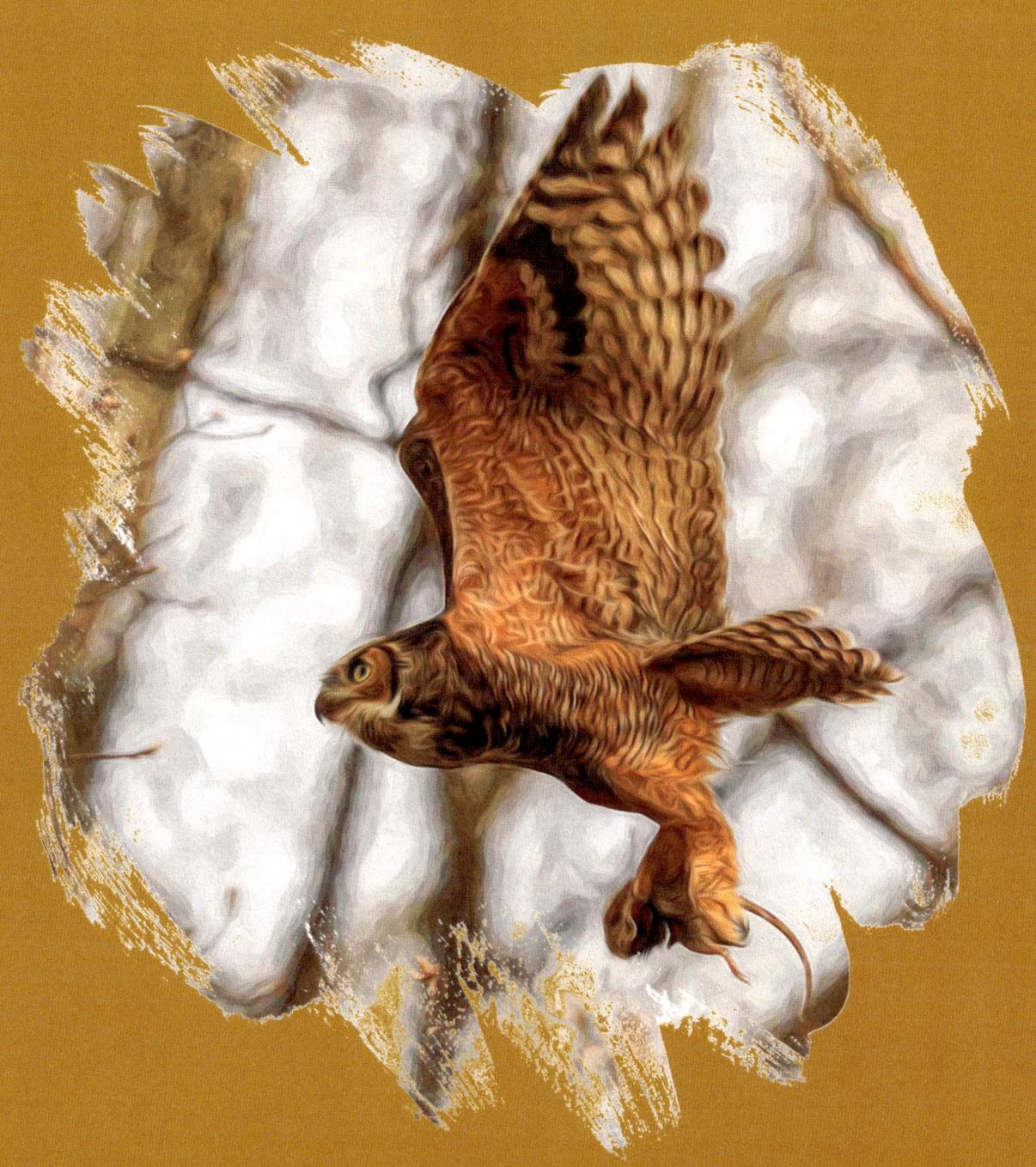

Each day brought growth and excitement. The owl parents took very good care of their little ones, high up in the tall pine tree in the small city forest.

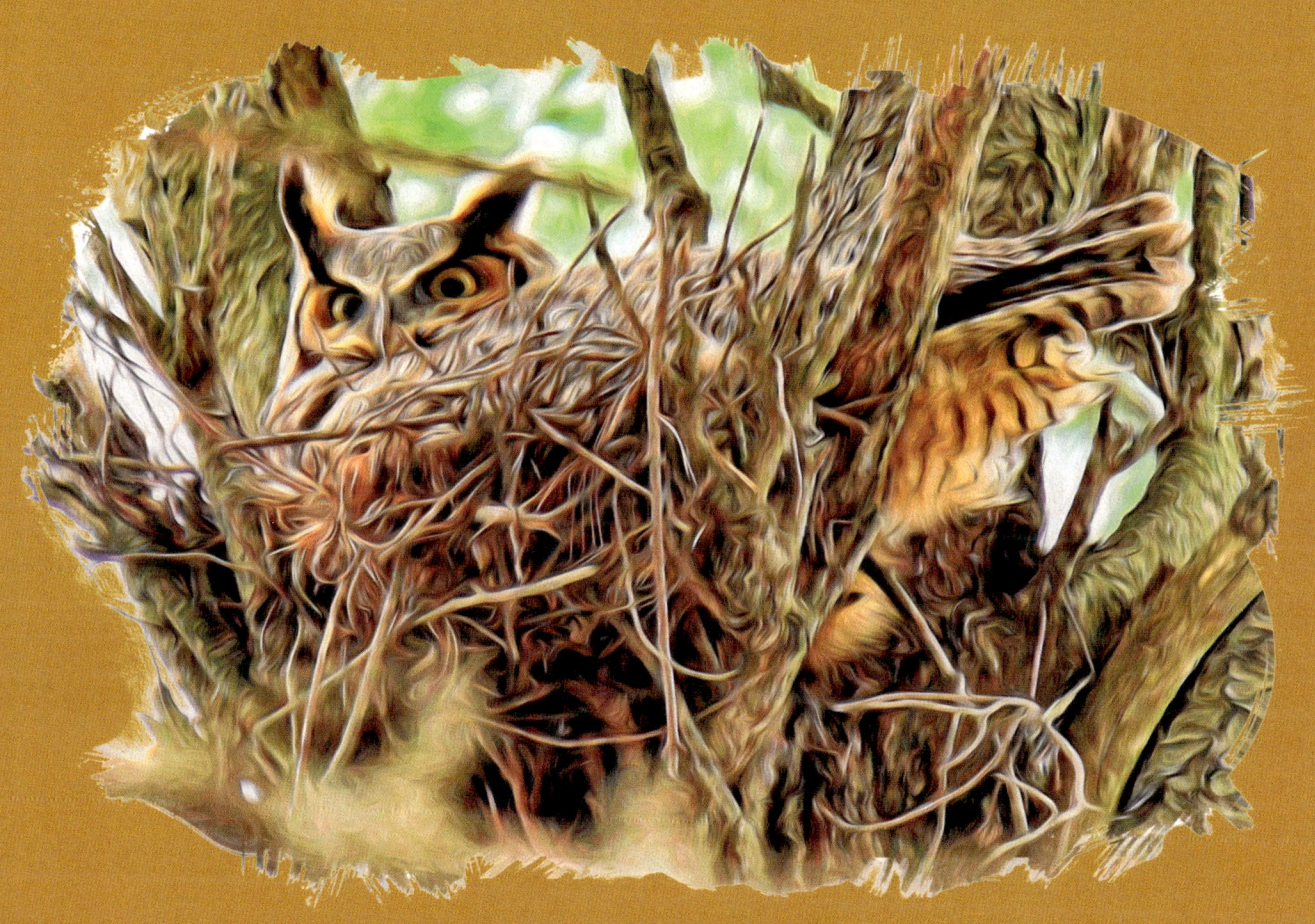

But one day, a sad thing happened. One owlet didn't wake up. No one was able to save it. The remaining owlet was now all alone.

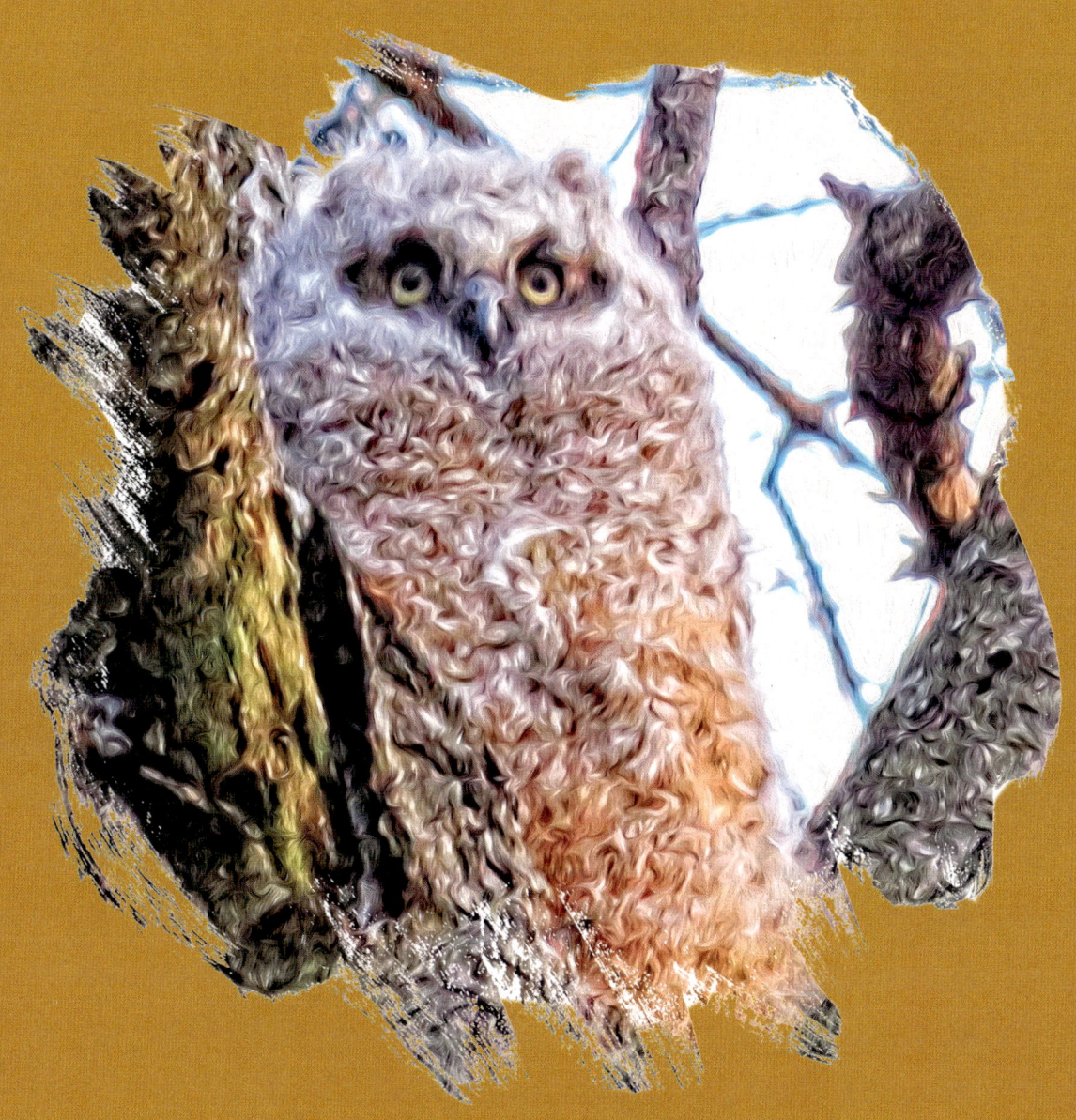

Now, the Owl parents had to give all their attention to their remaining owlet.

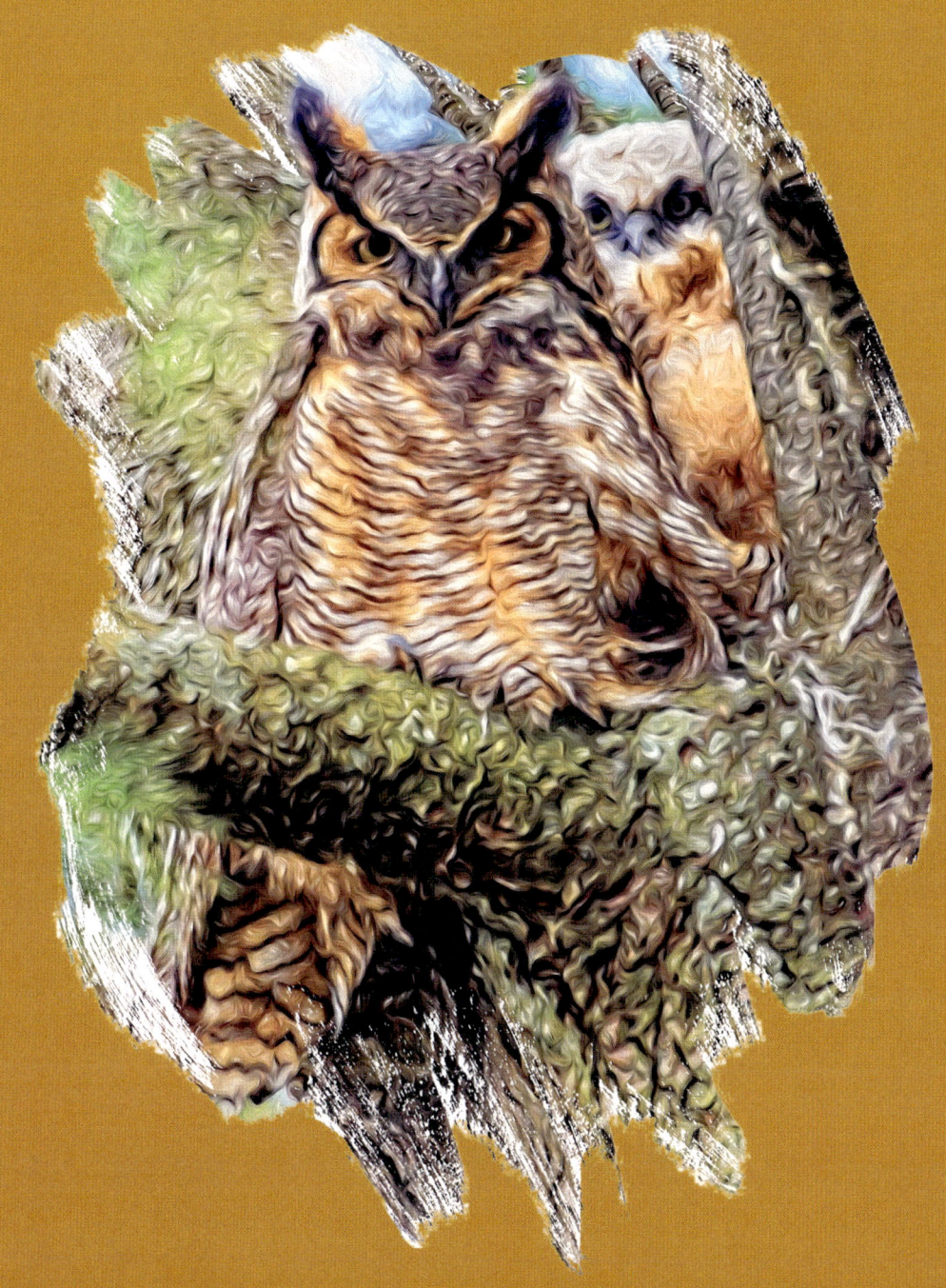

Time passed, which helped to heal the sadness of losing the other owlet.

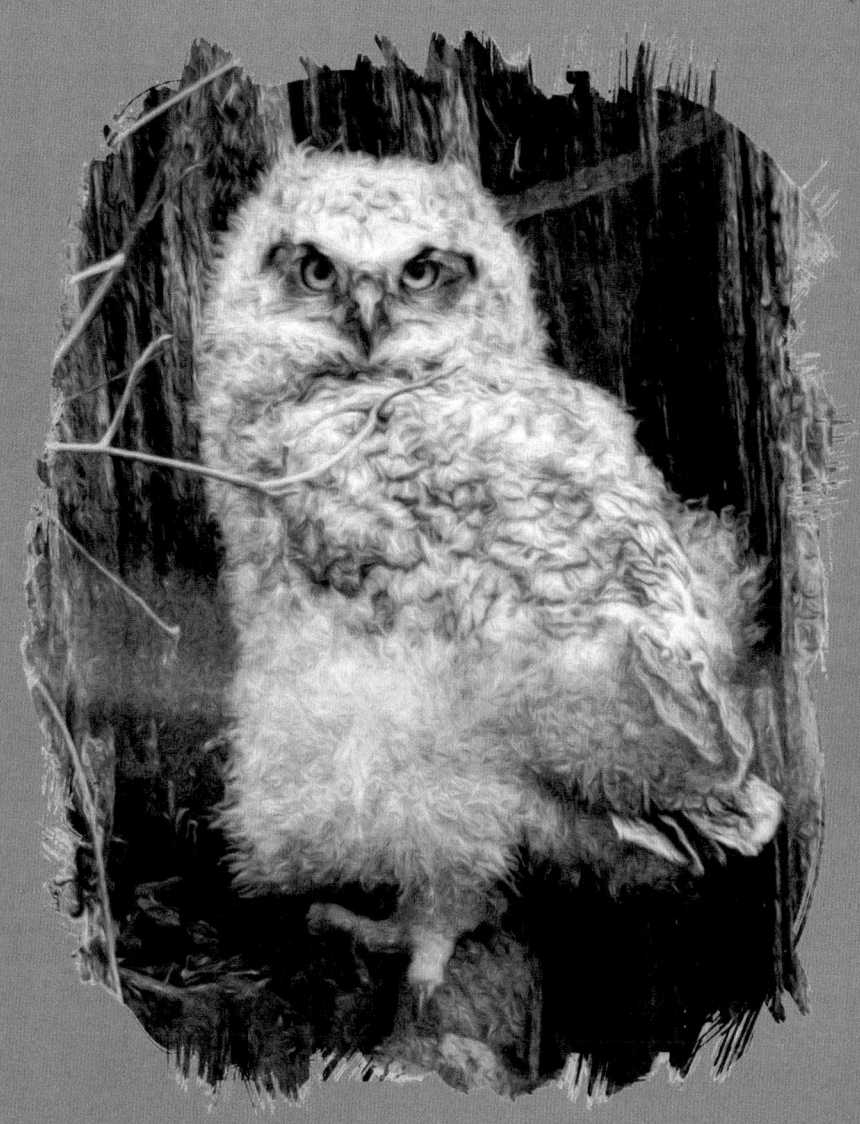

Mari was a young girl who liked to watch these owls. She suggested naming the owlet Skylar. We do not know if Skylar was a "he" or a "she," because it is very hard to know this when an owl is very young.

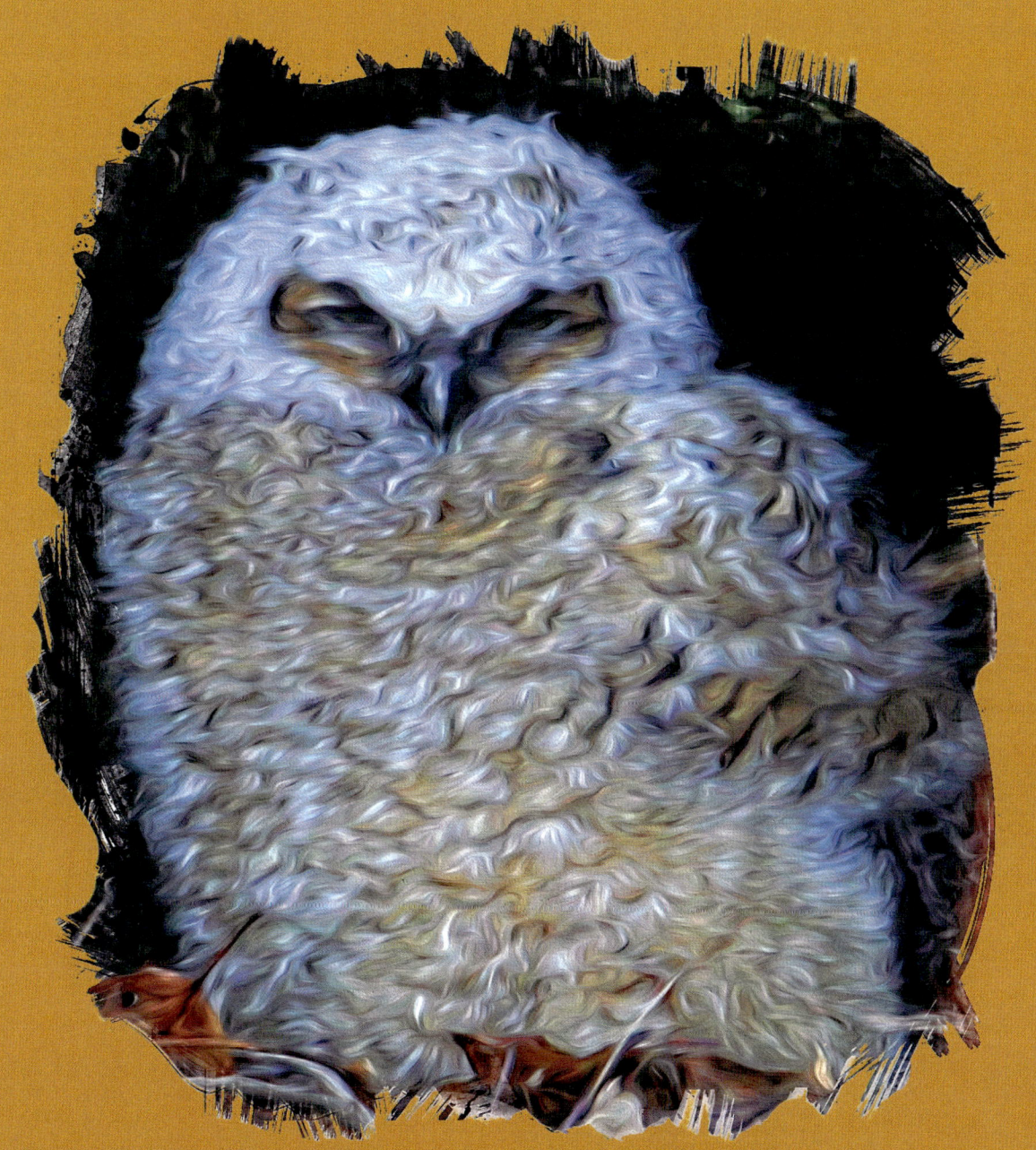

We will learn some things about Skylar even before Skylar learned them. Skylar was smart. Skylar was strong. And Skylar was a very lucky owlet!

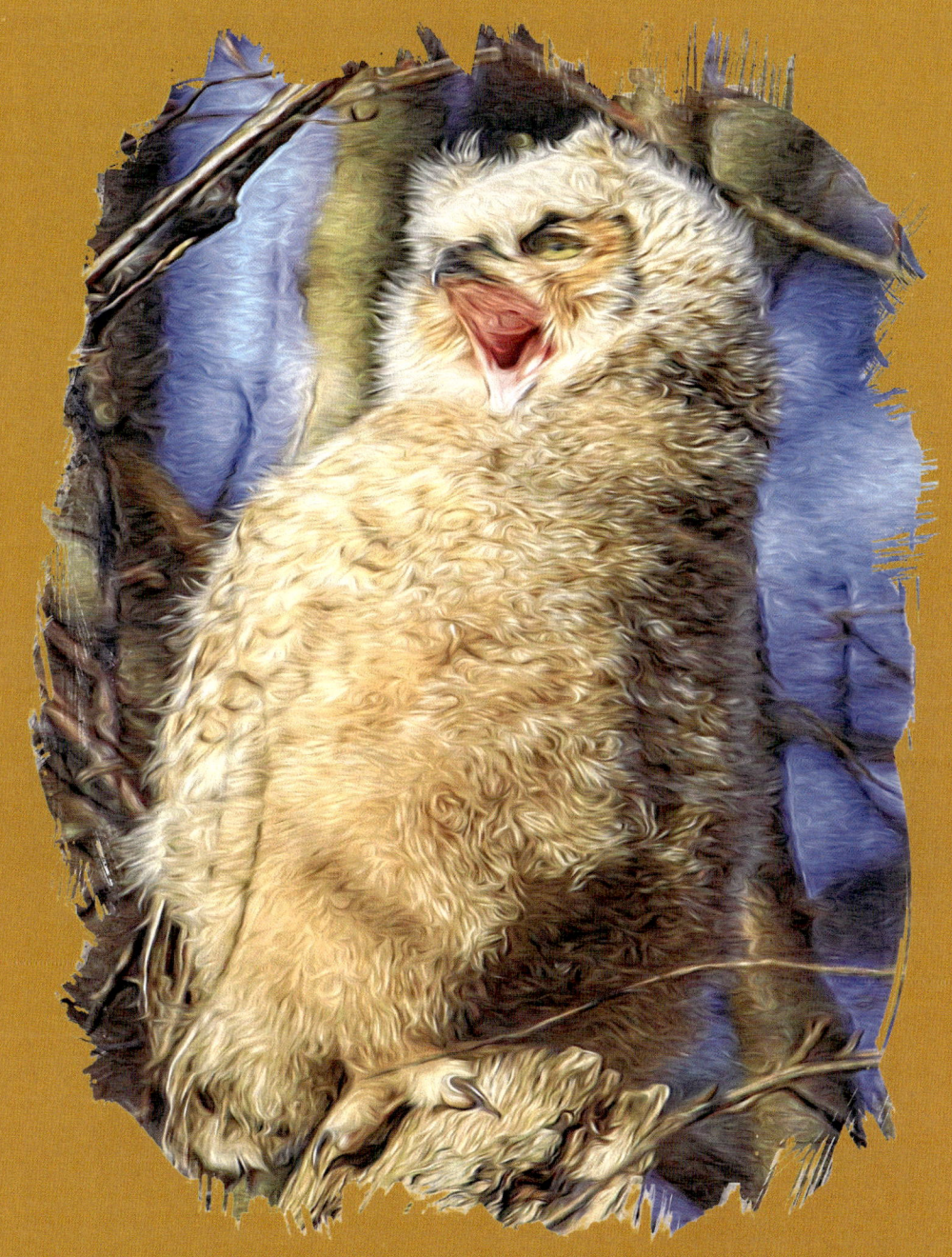

On April 12, Skylar took a misstep while branching, and fell out of the nest tree! Branching is what young owls do to get stronger when they leave the nest. It was a scary accident. How would Skylar survive such a fall?

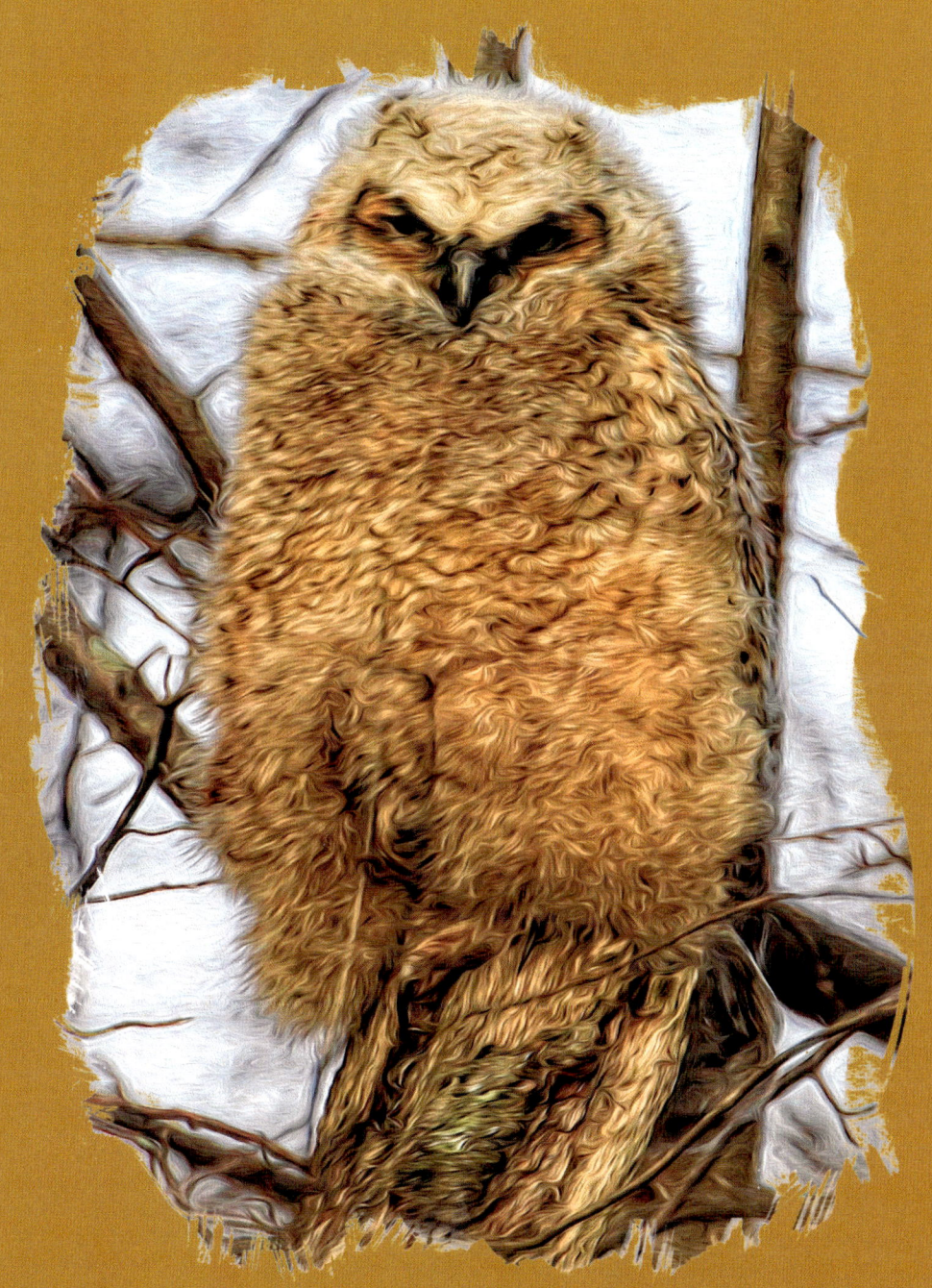

Skylar, you know by now, was a very special owl. The fall came so fast that Skylar just threw up its newly-feathered owl wings. The wings acted like a parachute, and Skylar landed gently on the ground. Skylar survived!

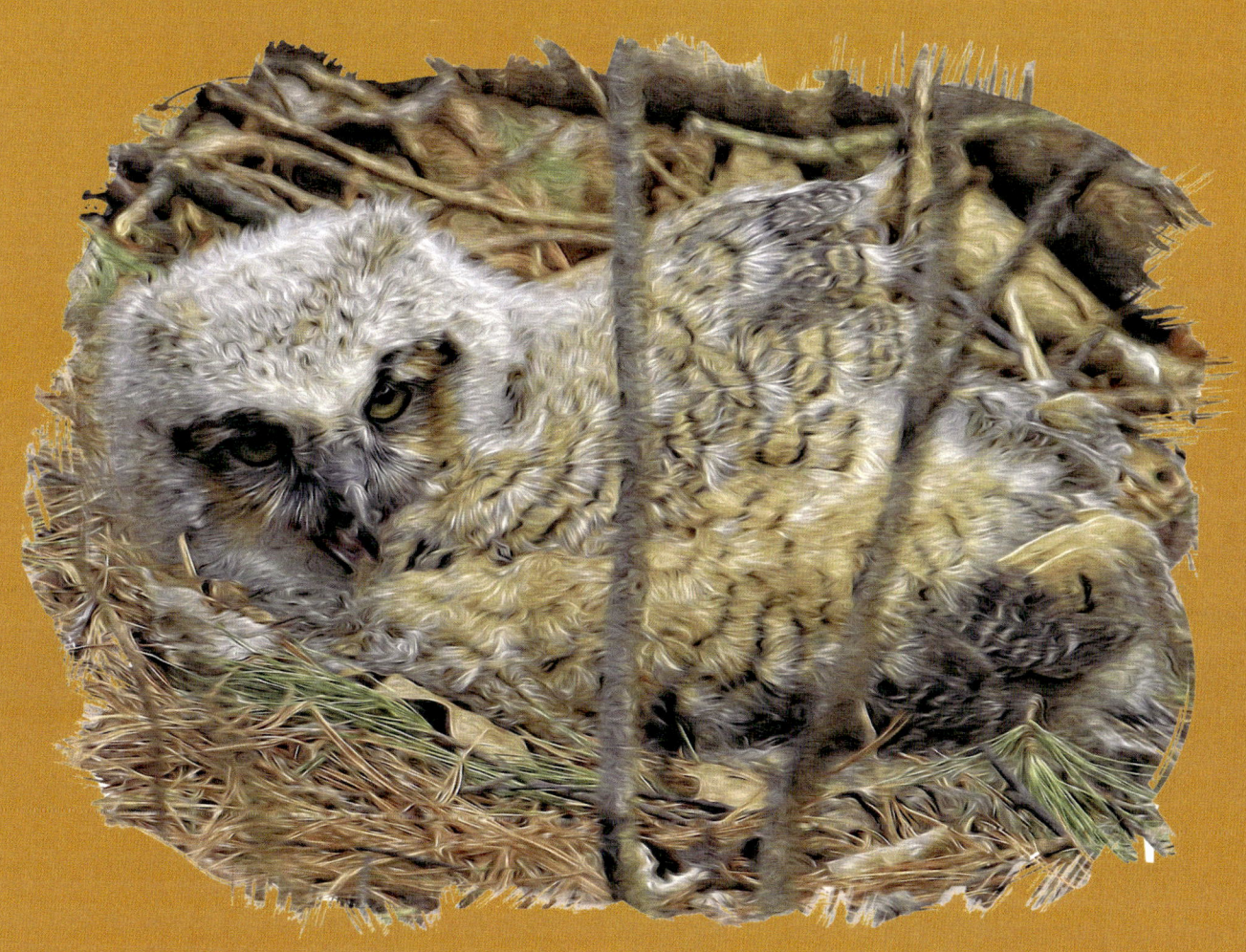

The Owl parents were so worried! Was the little owlet hurt? It was very dangerous for Skylar to be on the ground, without any defenses. There were many dangers for an unprepared young owlet that fell out of the tree.

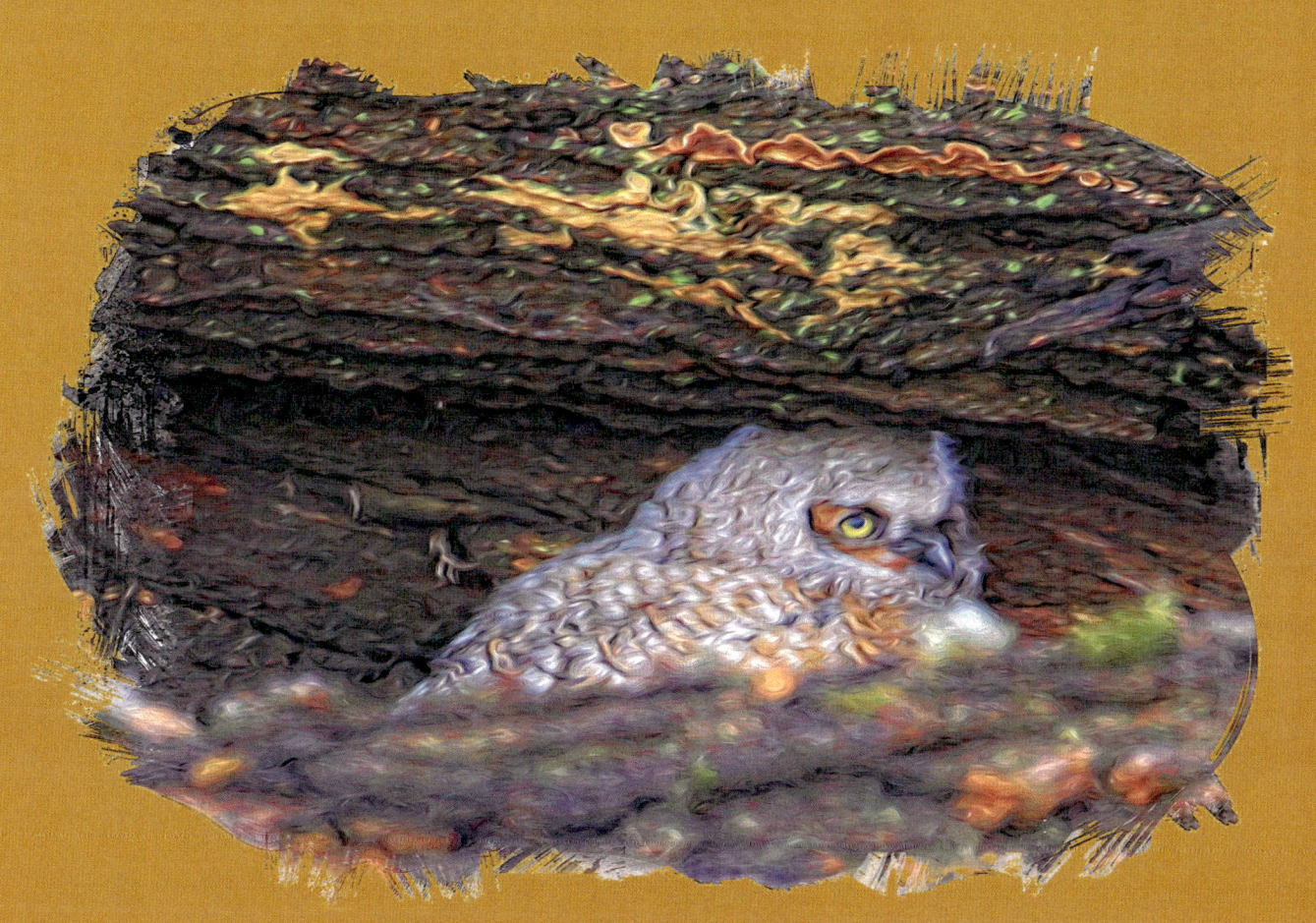

Owls need time in the nest to develop balance and strength. Walking out of the nest onto the branches trains them, and they need to do this for some time. But now, Skylar was on the ground alone without enough of this training.

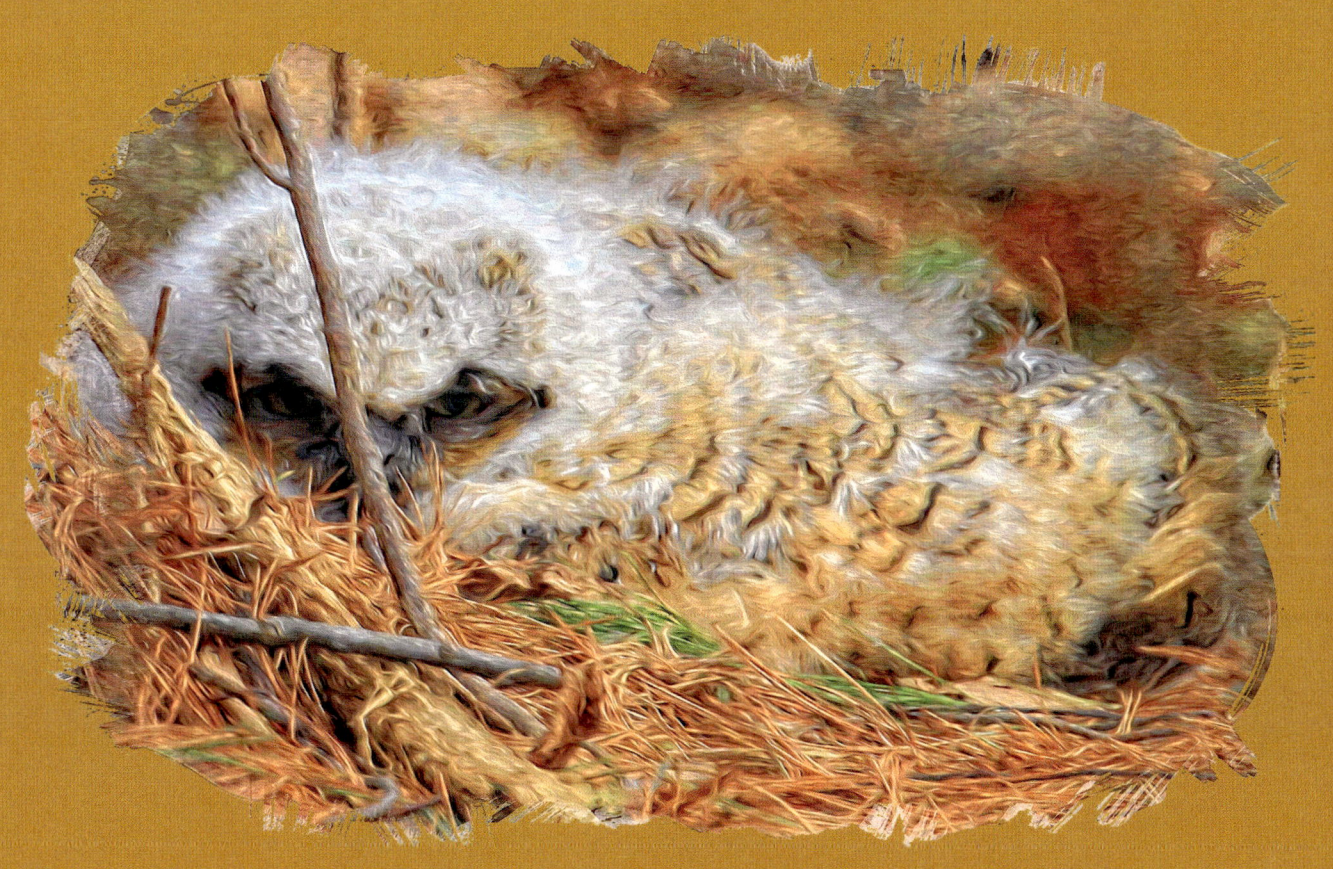

One morning, it began to rain very hard. It was turning out to be a very cold and wet Spring, and soon poor Skylar was a sopping mess.

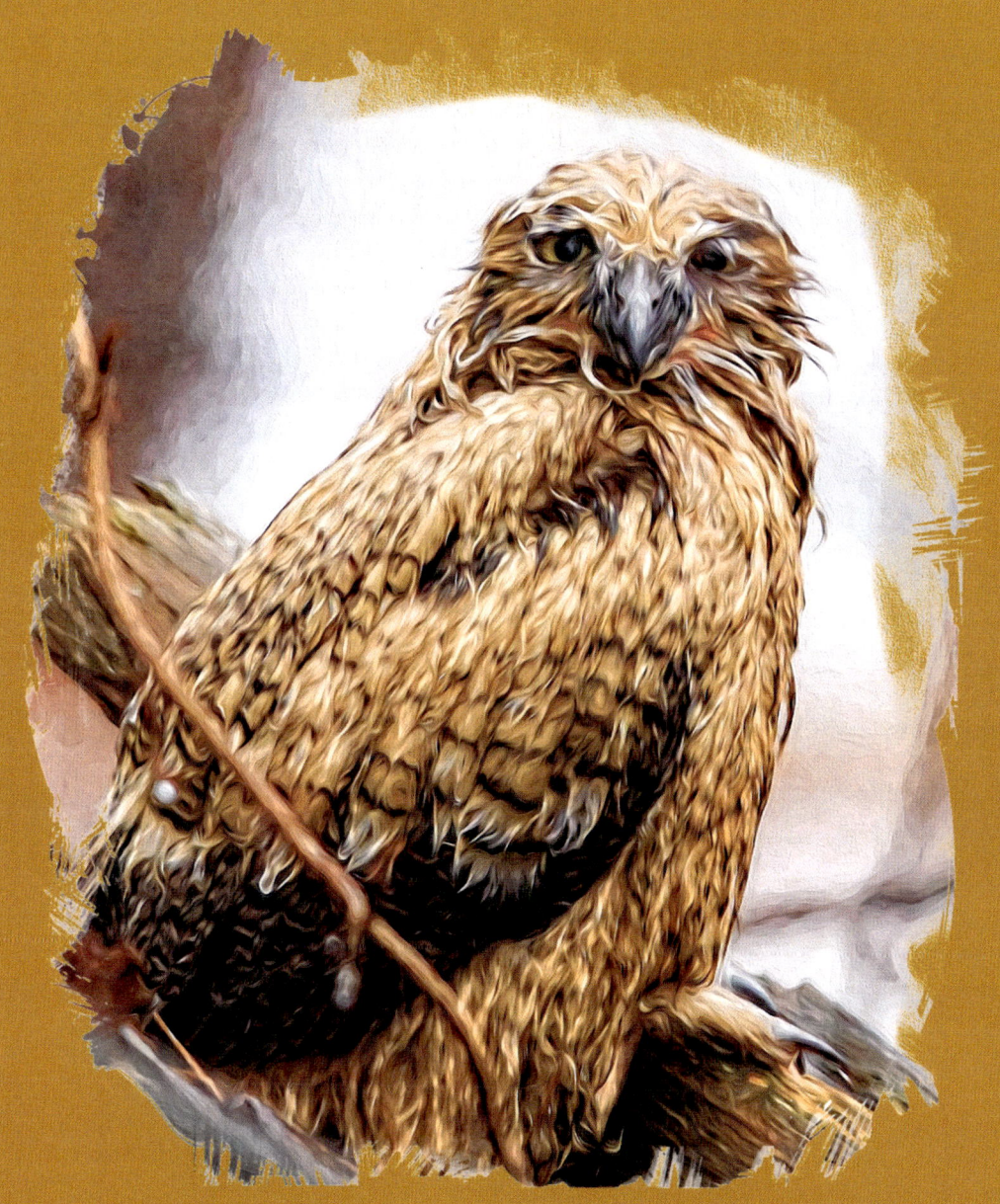

What do we know about Skylar? Skylar was smart. Skylar was strong. Skylar was very lucky!

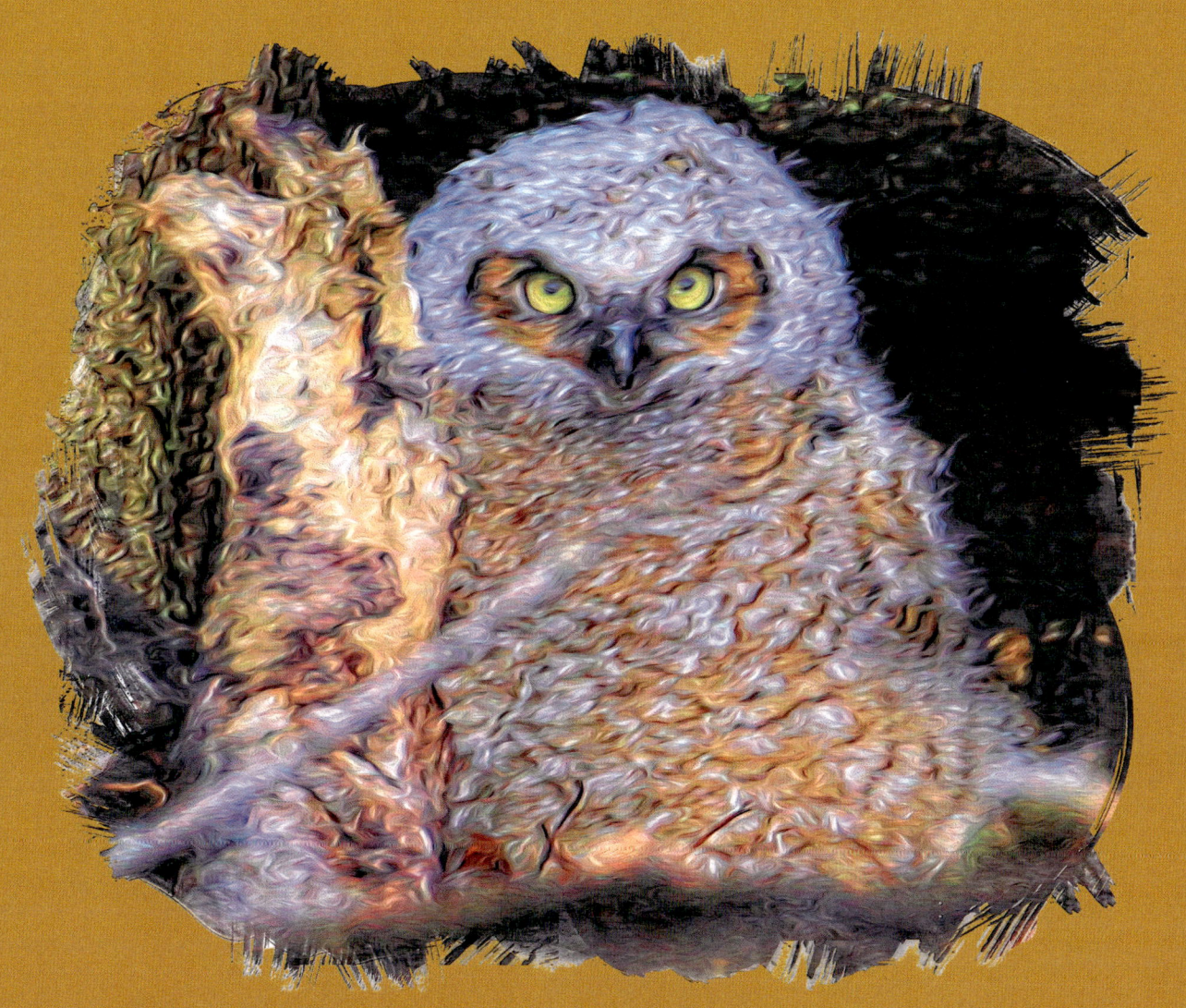

Skylar stayed silent on the ground. You didn't want to attract attention to yourself if you were an owlet that fell out of the tree!

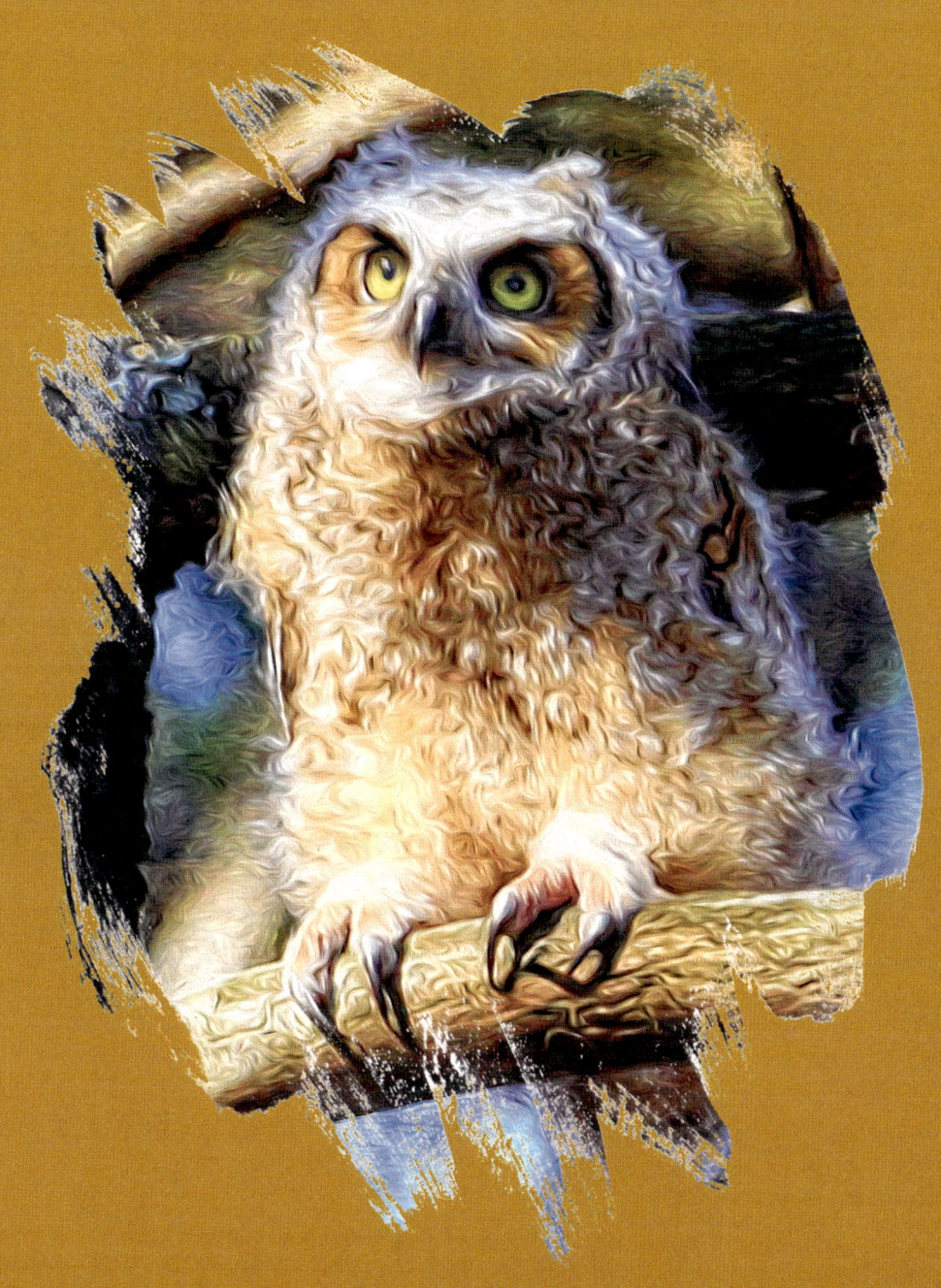

That first night was very scary. At night, the small city forest filled with strange animal noises, and Skylar was alone and cold, too weak to move off of the ground.

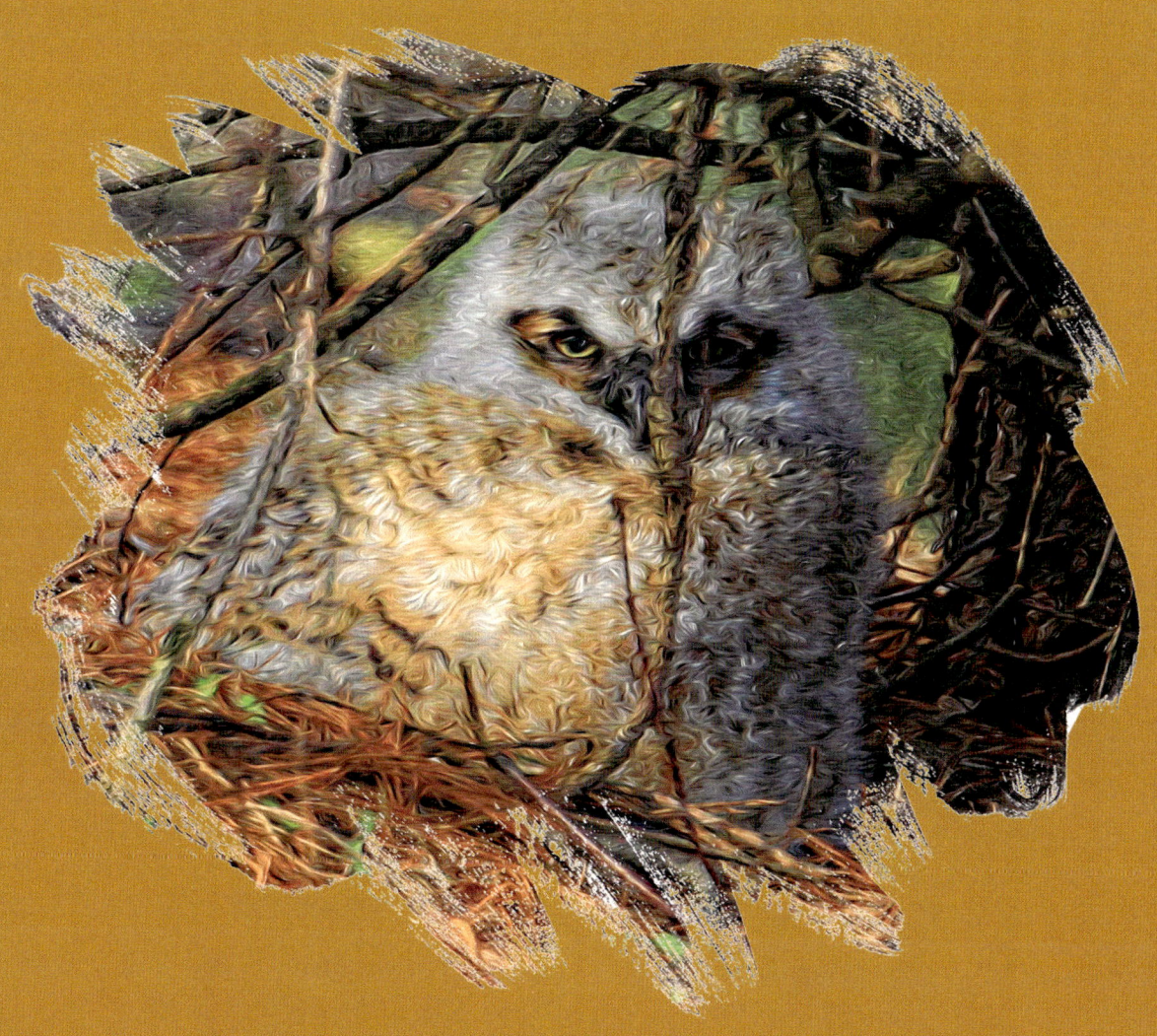

But the owlet wasn't totally alone. The Mother and Father Owl were always nearby. They brought food to Skylar, and Skylar gained strength.

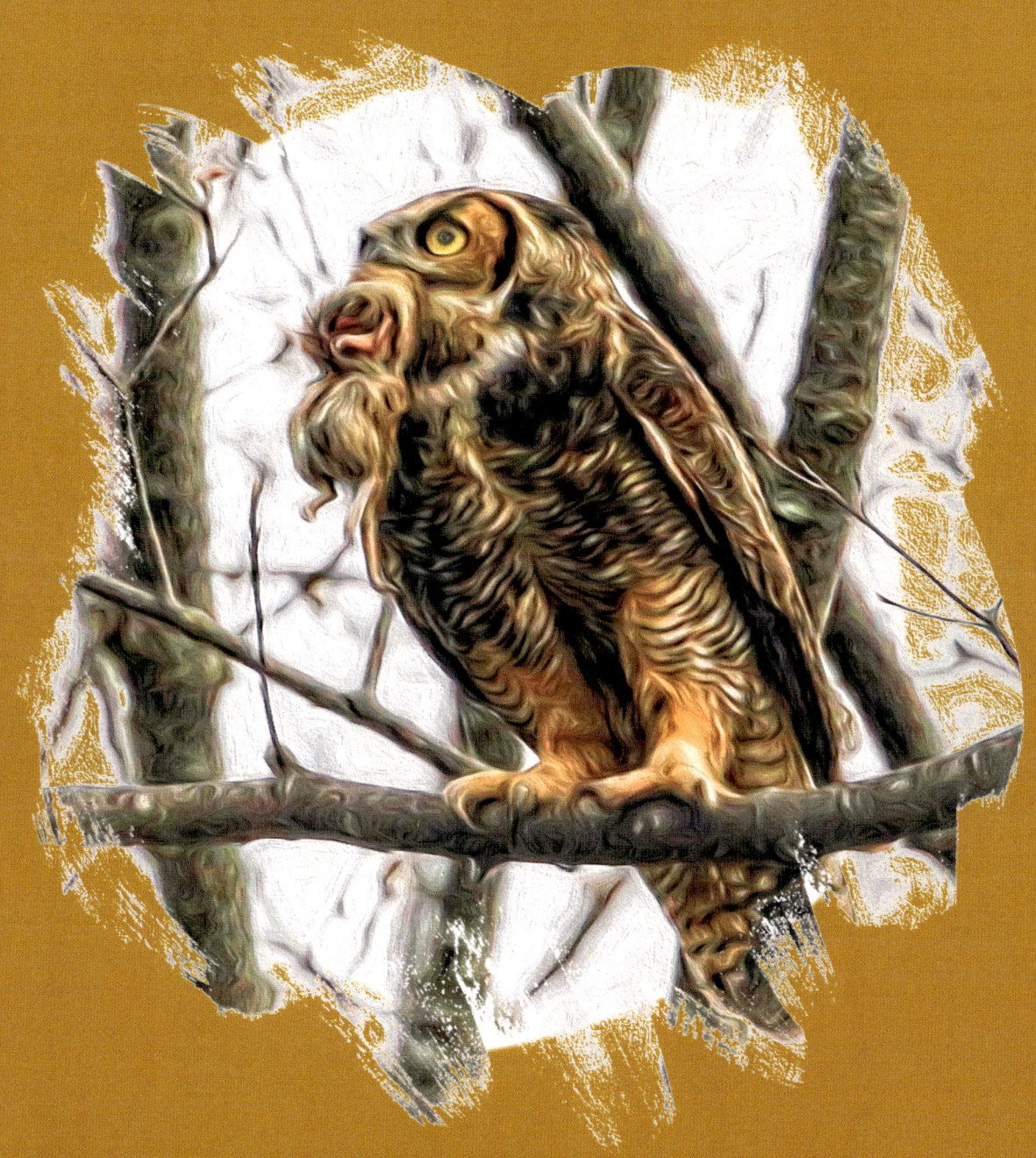

43

The owl's human friends also helped. When they discovered the little owlet that had fallen out of the tree, someone put "CAUTION" tape around the area near Skylar, so people wouldn't get too close and scare Skylar. The Park Rangers placed signs along the path telling people about the owlet and asking dog walkers to keep their dogs leashed. These things helped Skylar stay safe.

GROUNDED BABY OWL AHEAD

PLEASE

PUT DOGS ON LEASH AND RESPECT FENCING

Skylar's human friends didn't help the owlet get back to its nest because the owl parents wouldn't allow it. Skylar had to do this alone.

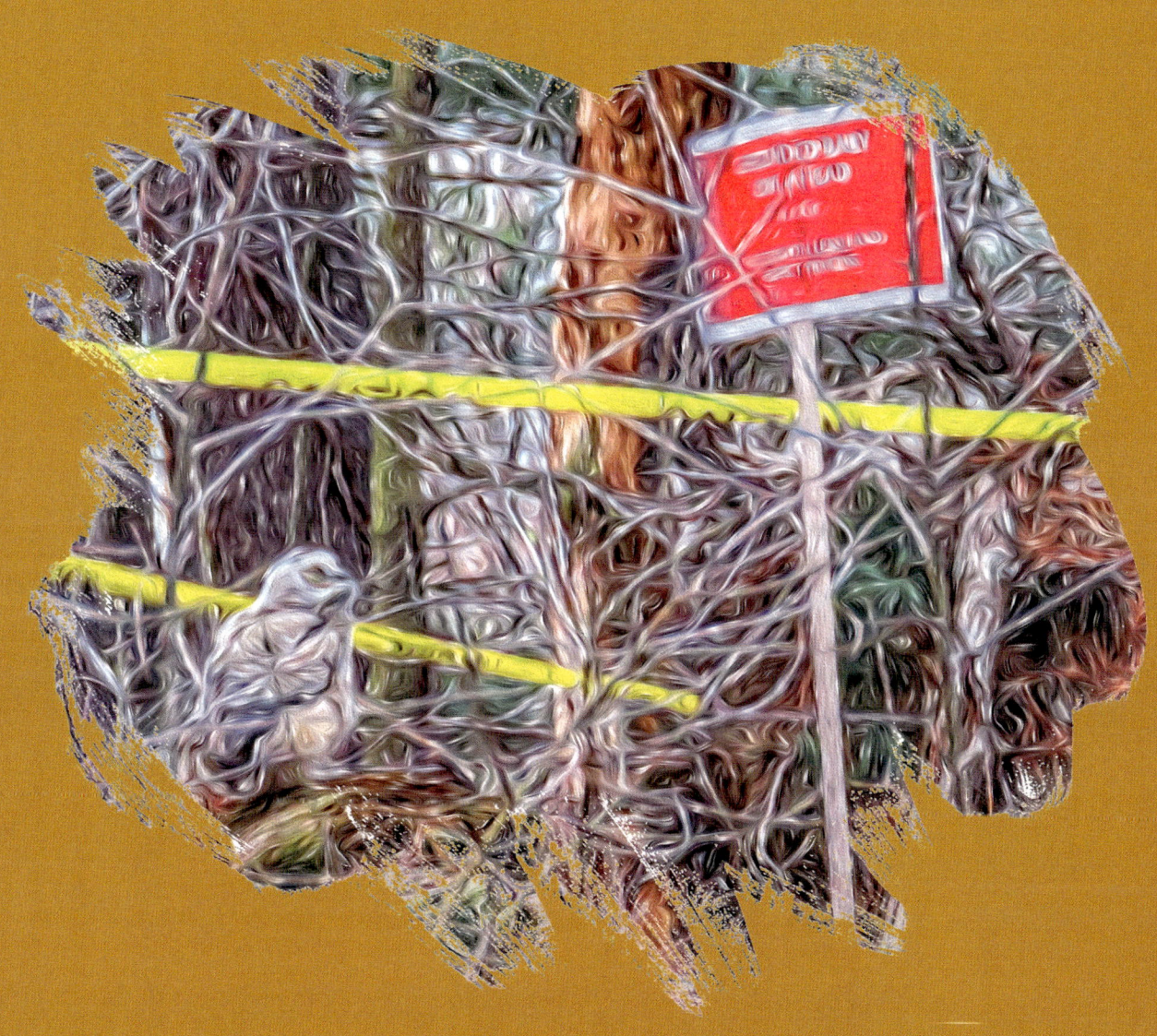

47

Skylar was often afraid, but the Mother and Father Owl hooted sounds of encouragement. Each day Skylar was able to move a bit more, and soon was strong enough to climb small forest limbs and bent branches to get off the ground.

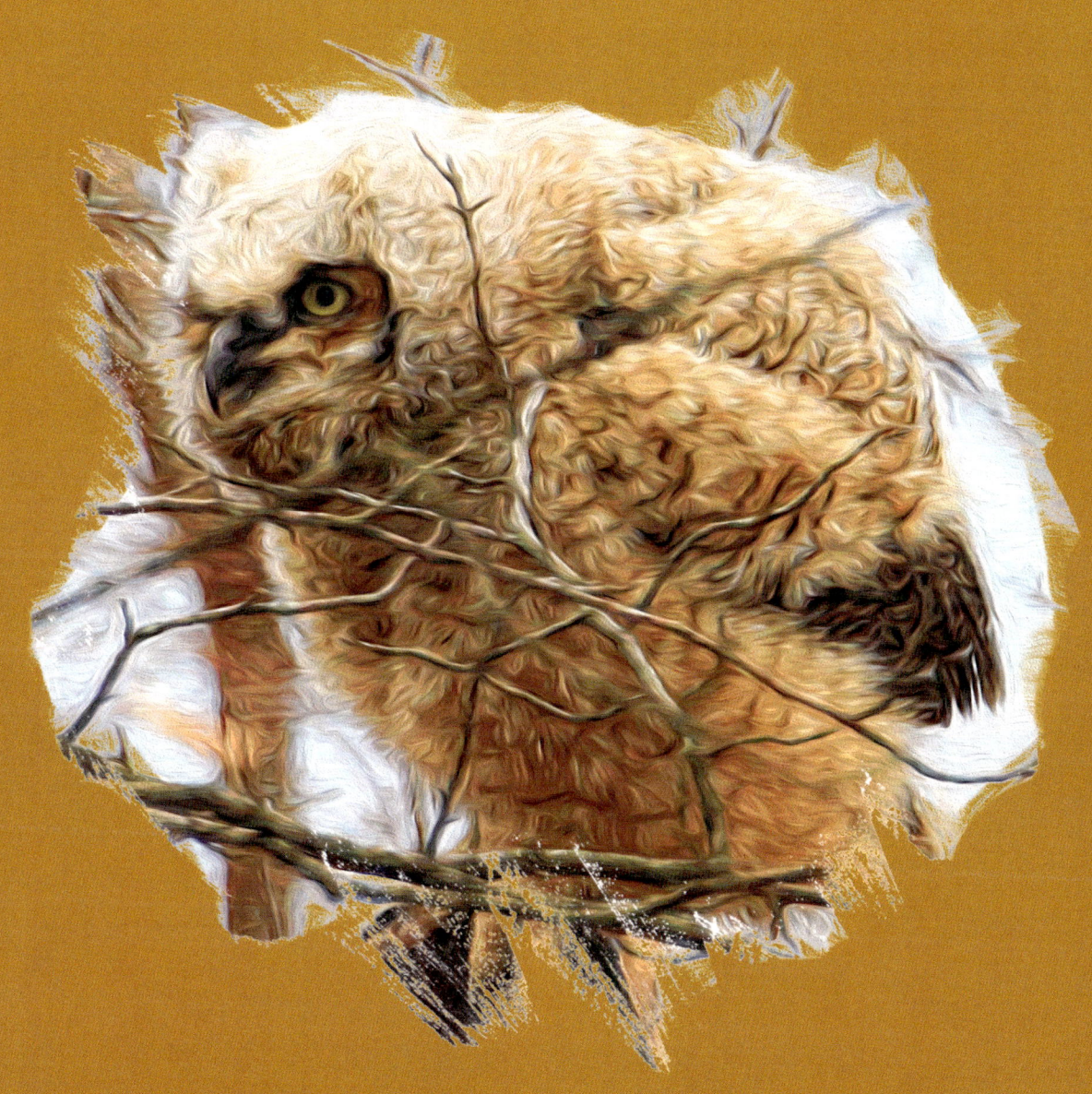

Over the course of several days, the little owlet climbed higher and higher, and this made Skylar stronger and stronger. Soon the little owlet was high enough to sit next to Mother Owl. She rubbed beaks with Skylar, and nuzzled her owlet, showing Skylar what a special and strong owl Skylar was. That made Skylar feel so good!

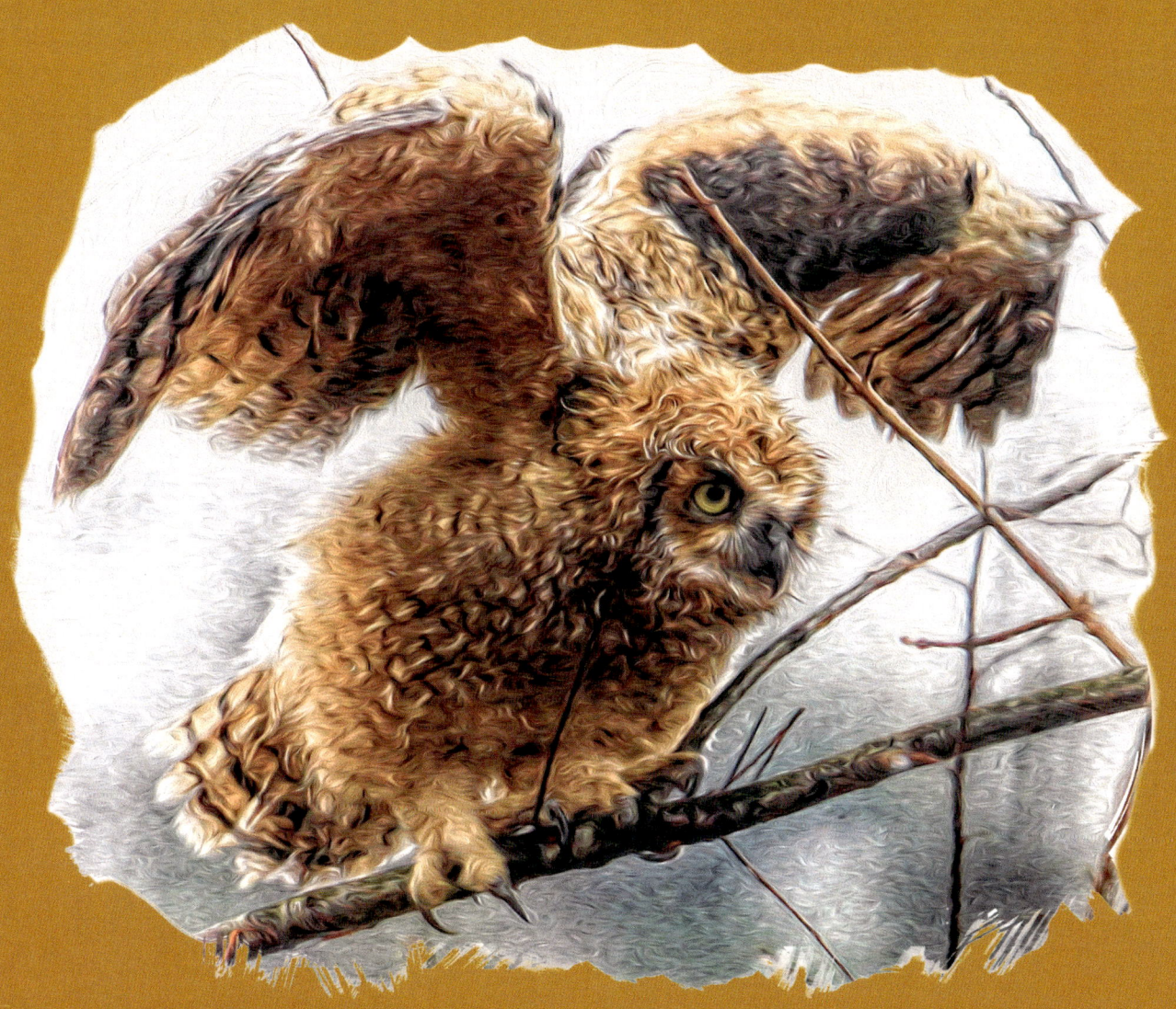

The owl's human friends came every day to watch Skylar's progress. Many of the humans were photographers who liked to take pictures of the owl family. The humans loved the owls, too.

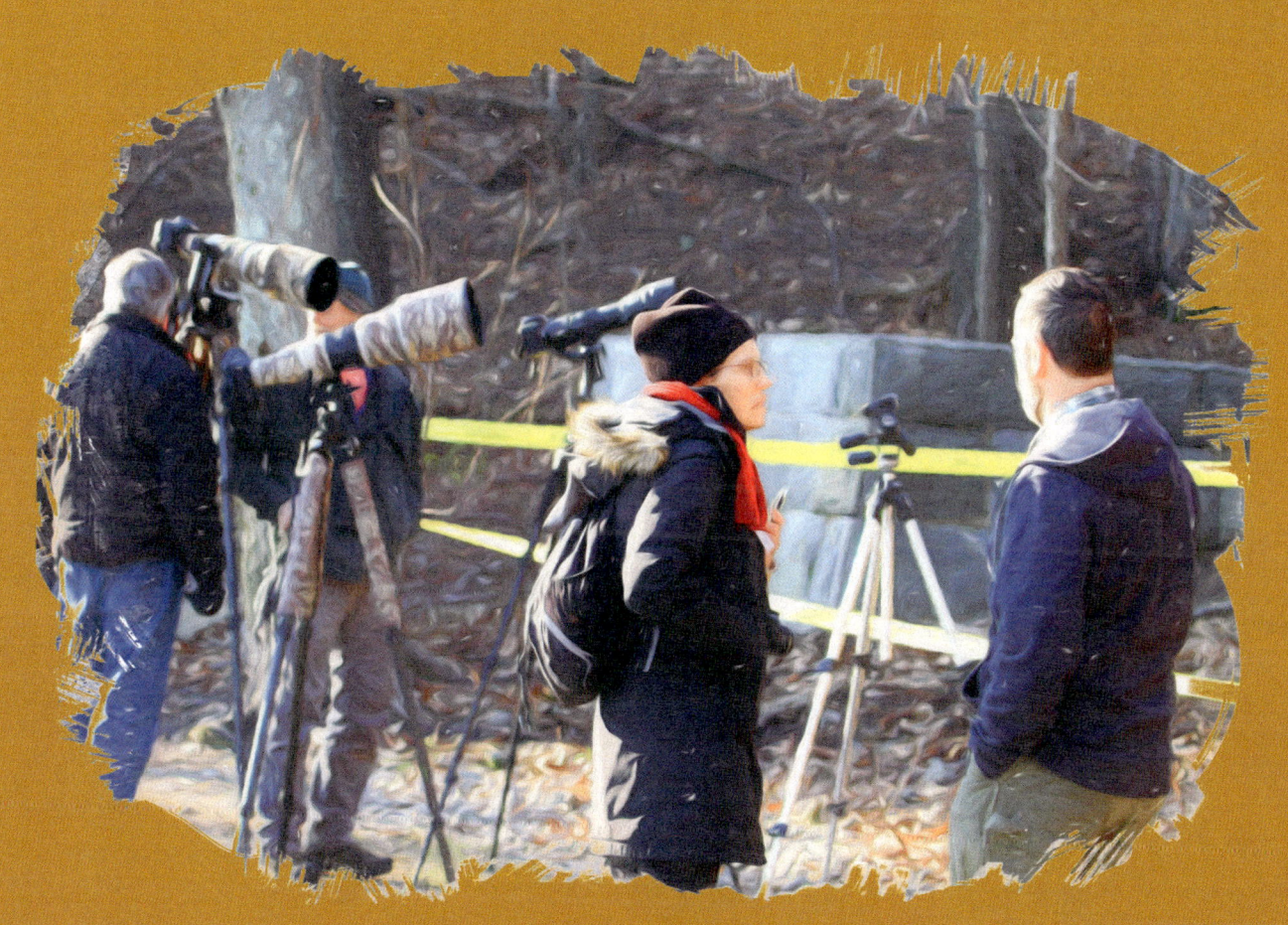

Skylar watched Mother and Father fly. Could Skylar fly? It looked so hard. And scary! Sometimes Skylar stretched and flapped, but still couldn't leave the perch. How did you do it? How did Skylar learn to fly?

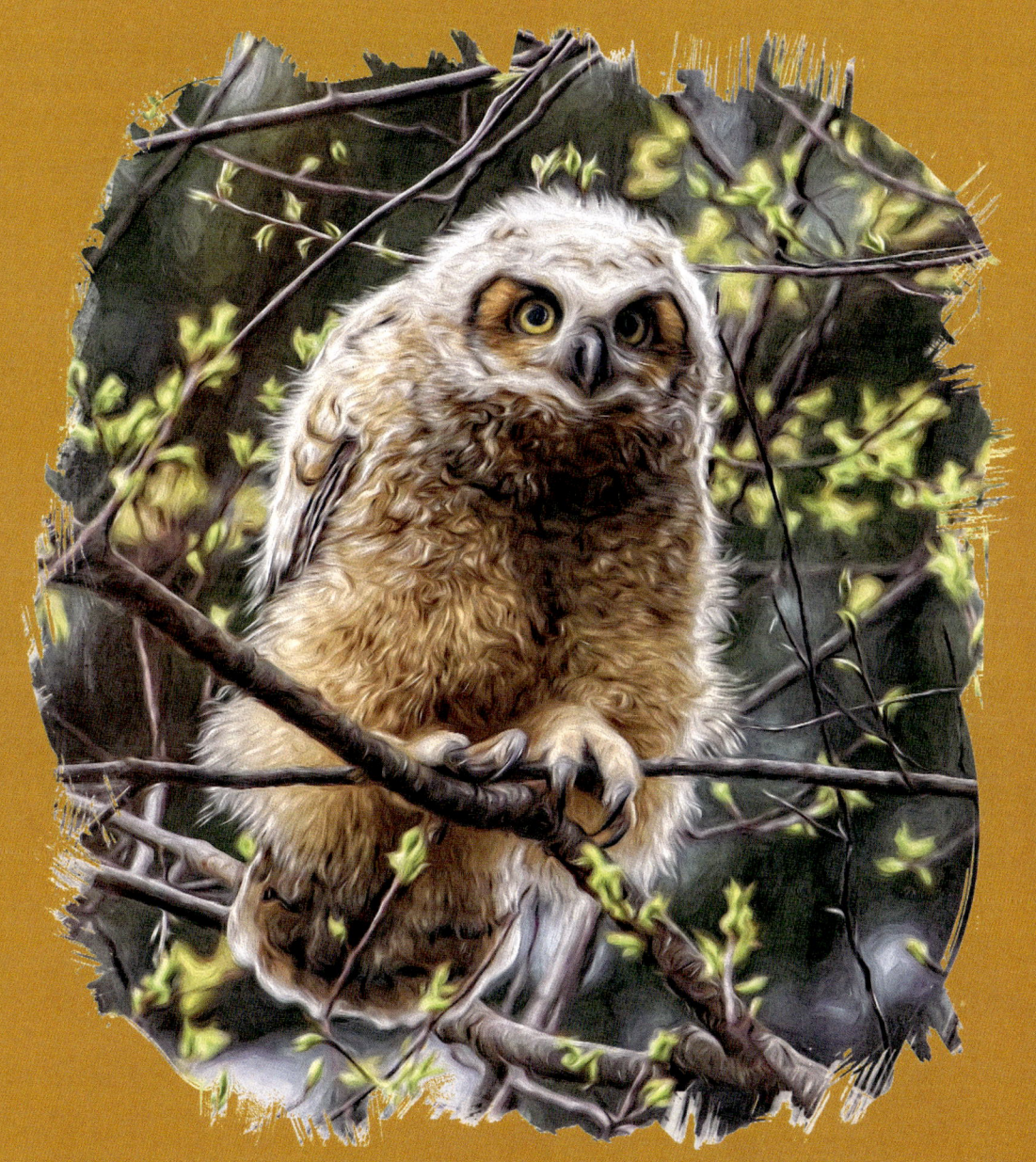

Well, all baby birds know how to fly; they just have to realize they can. They are made to fly and to live in the air. But, they have to Practice. They have to work hard. They have to be persistent. And one day, after all that, they fly.

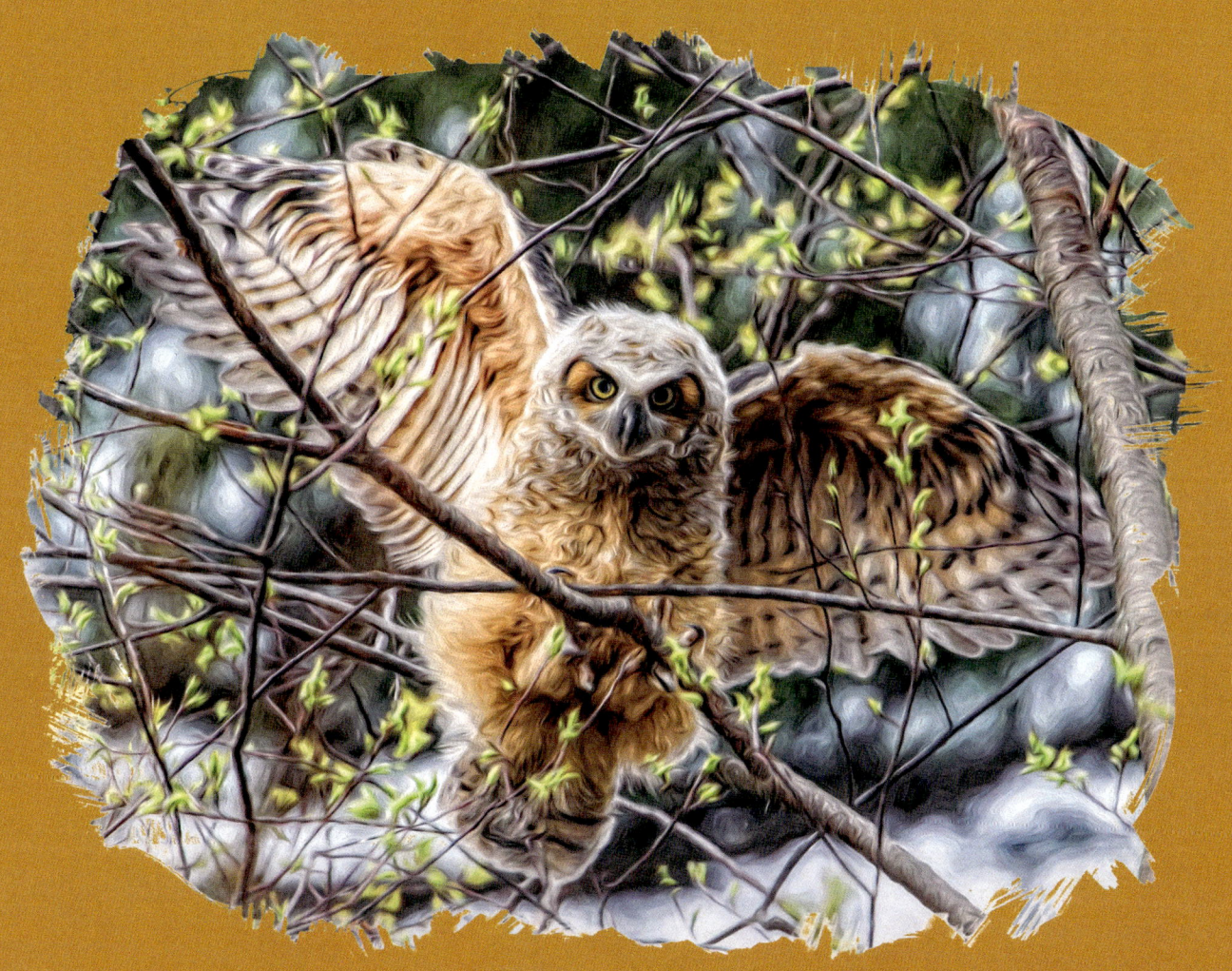

Saturday, April 28 was a special day for Skylar. After thinking about flying for so long, Skylar decided to do it. Skylar gathered up courage, looked at a branch to fly to, jumped high, and was actually airborne. Skylar made it to the other branch. Skylar flew!

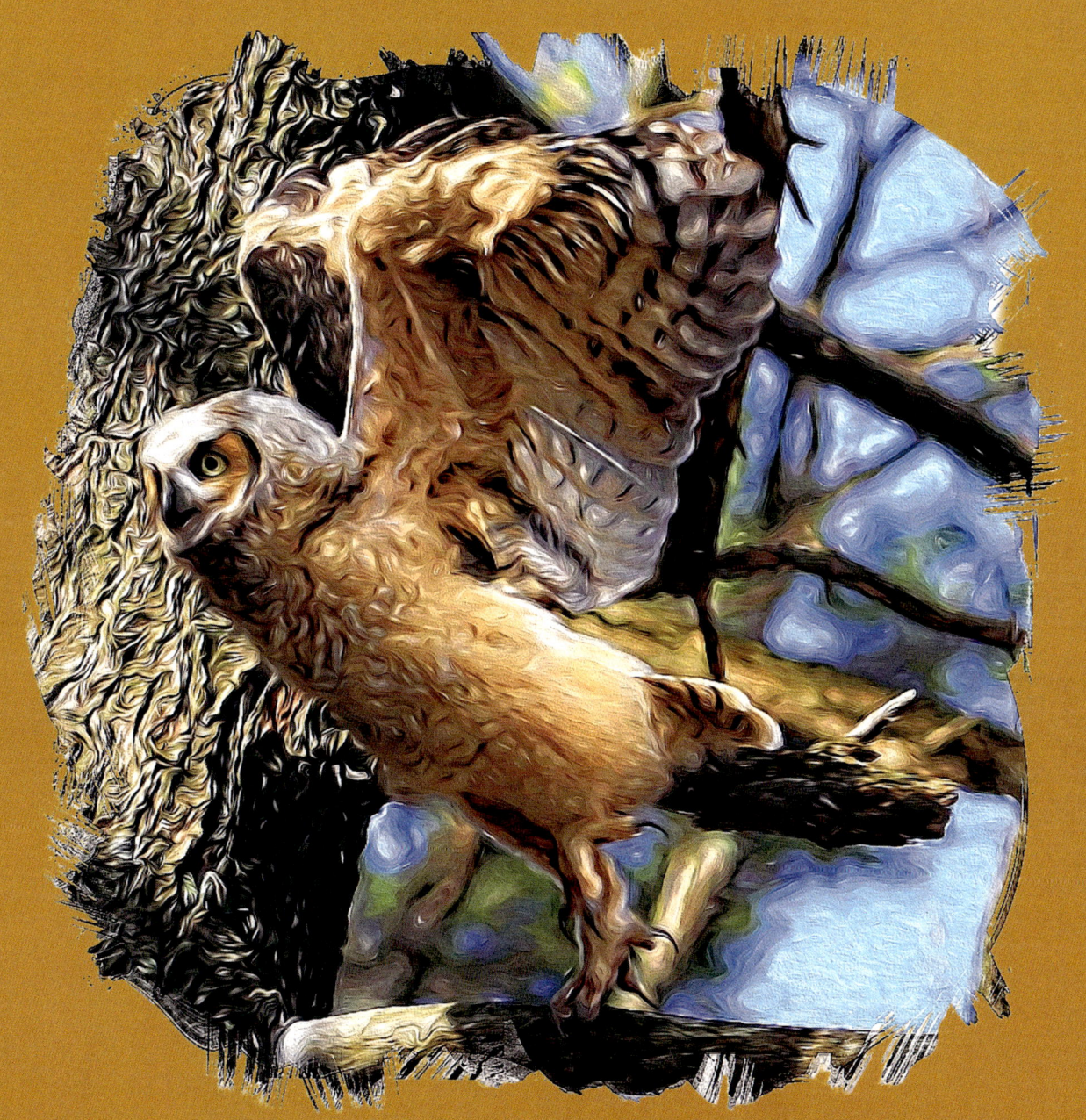

It was so exciting. The people below were so happy for the owlet. They took pictures, and some even clapped!

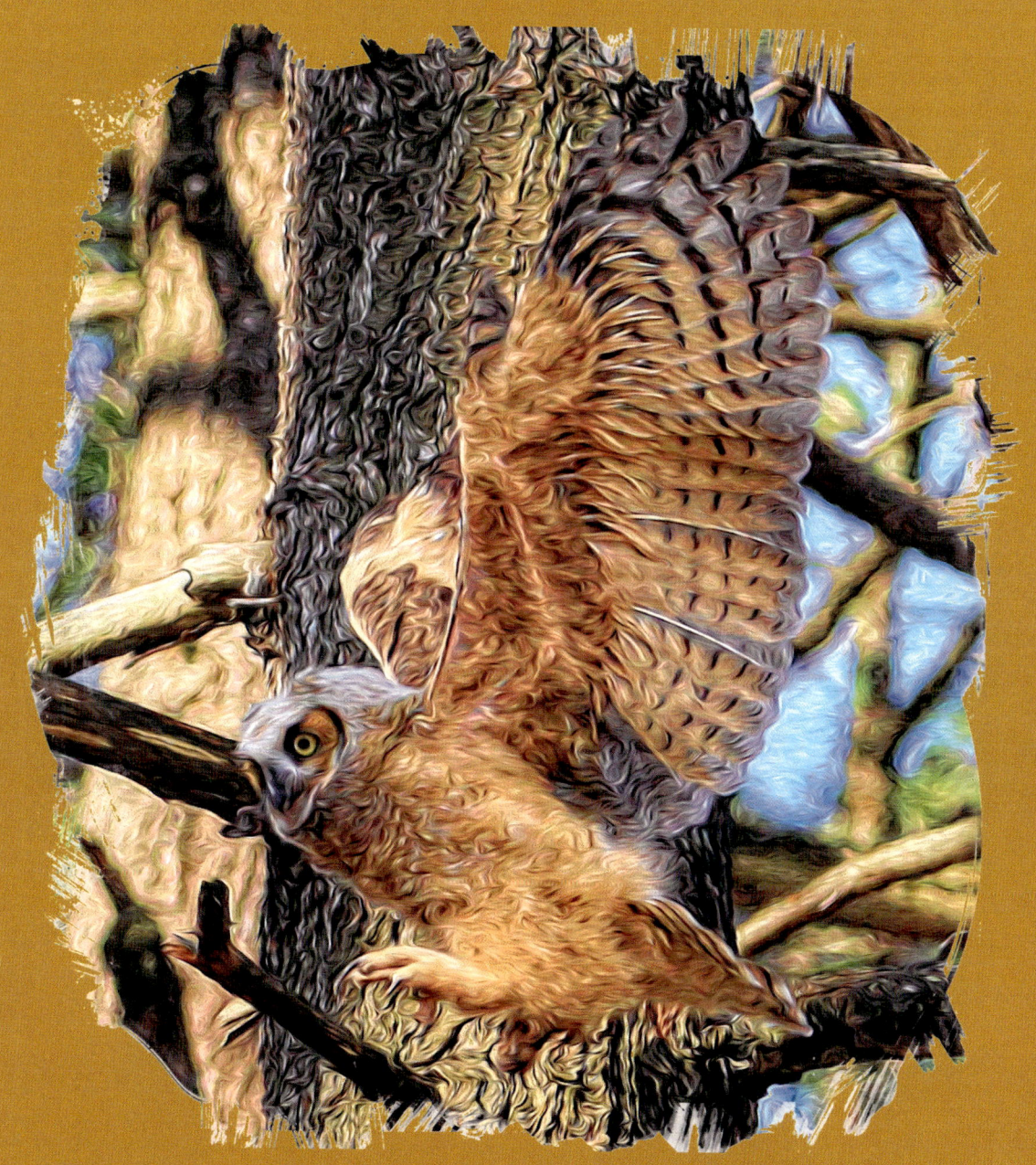

Skylar was growing up. The rest of that special Saturday was spent flying short distances, with Mother and Father watching Skylar, which encouraged the little owlet to keep it up.

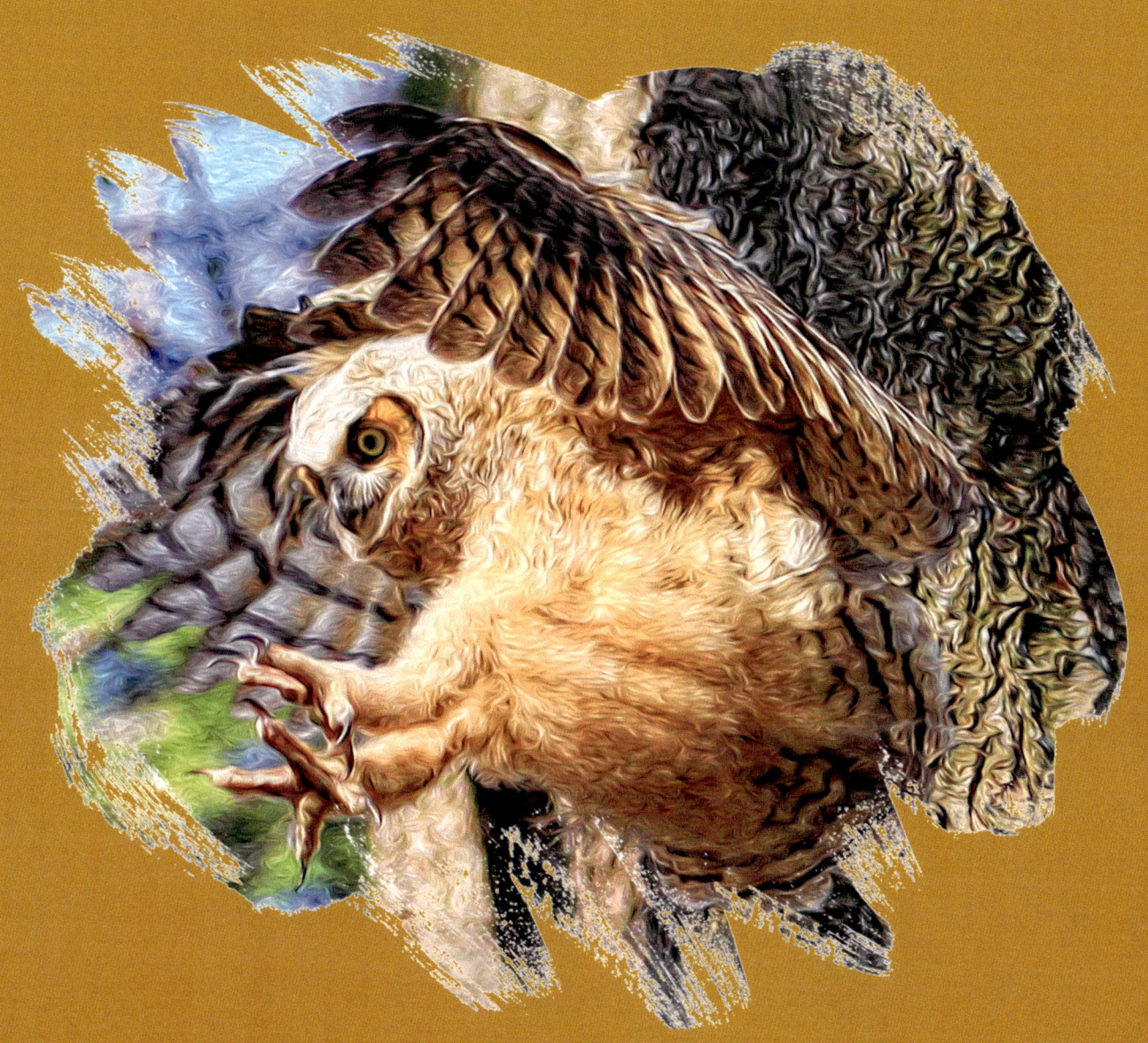

Owls take a long time to develop, and even though Skylar could now fly, there was still much to learn. Skylar knew to watch Mother and Father, for they had much to teach.

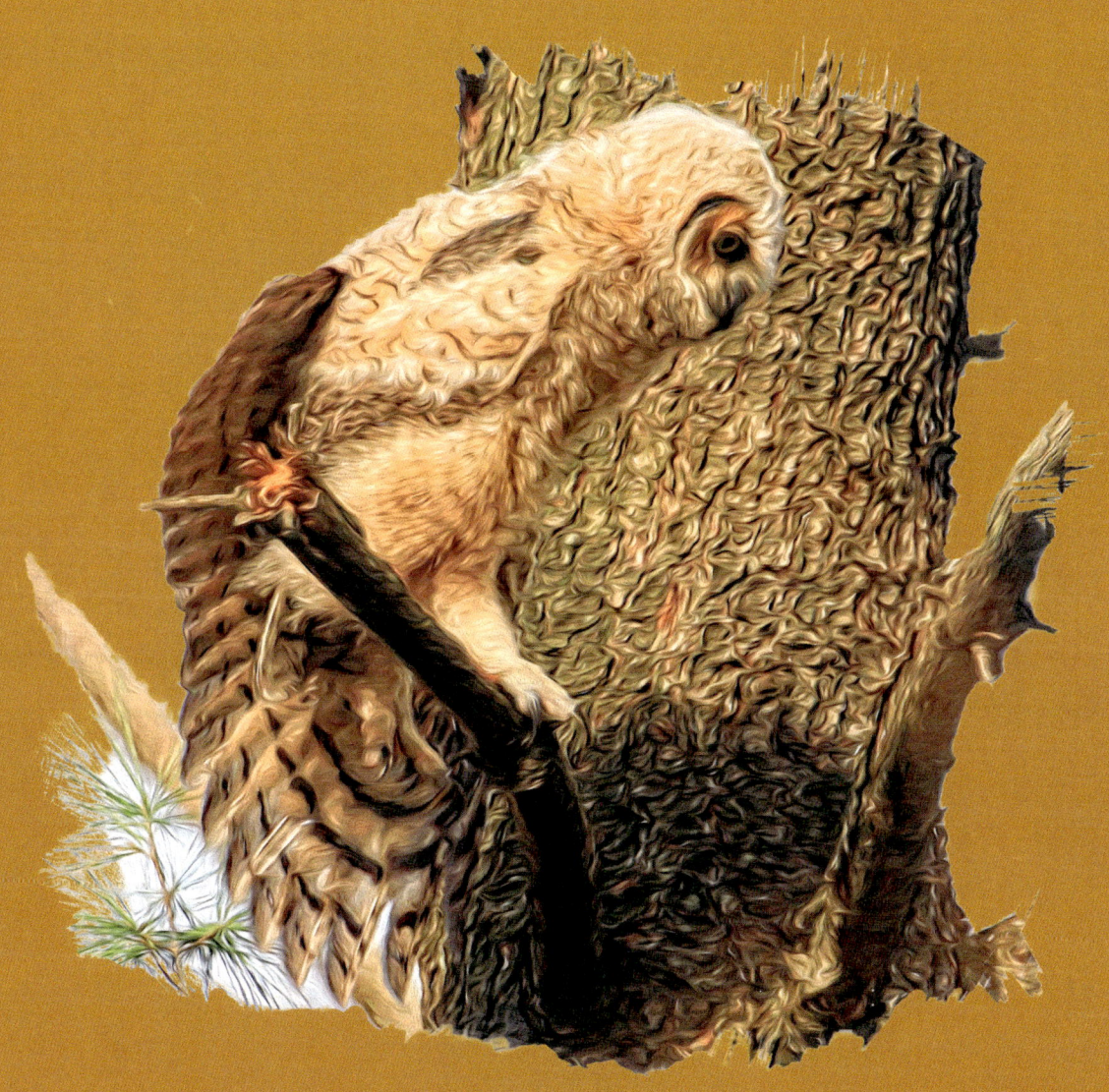

Each day, it got harder for the owl's human friends to see Skylar, because the owlet went higher and higher into the trees. Now, Skylar could really learn how to become a Great Horned Owl!

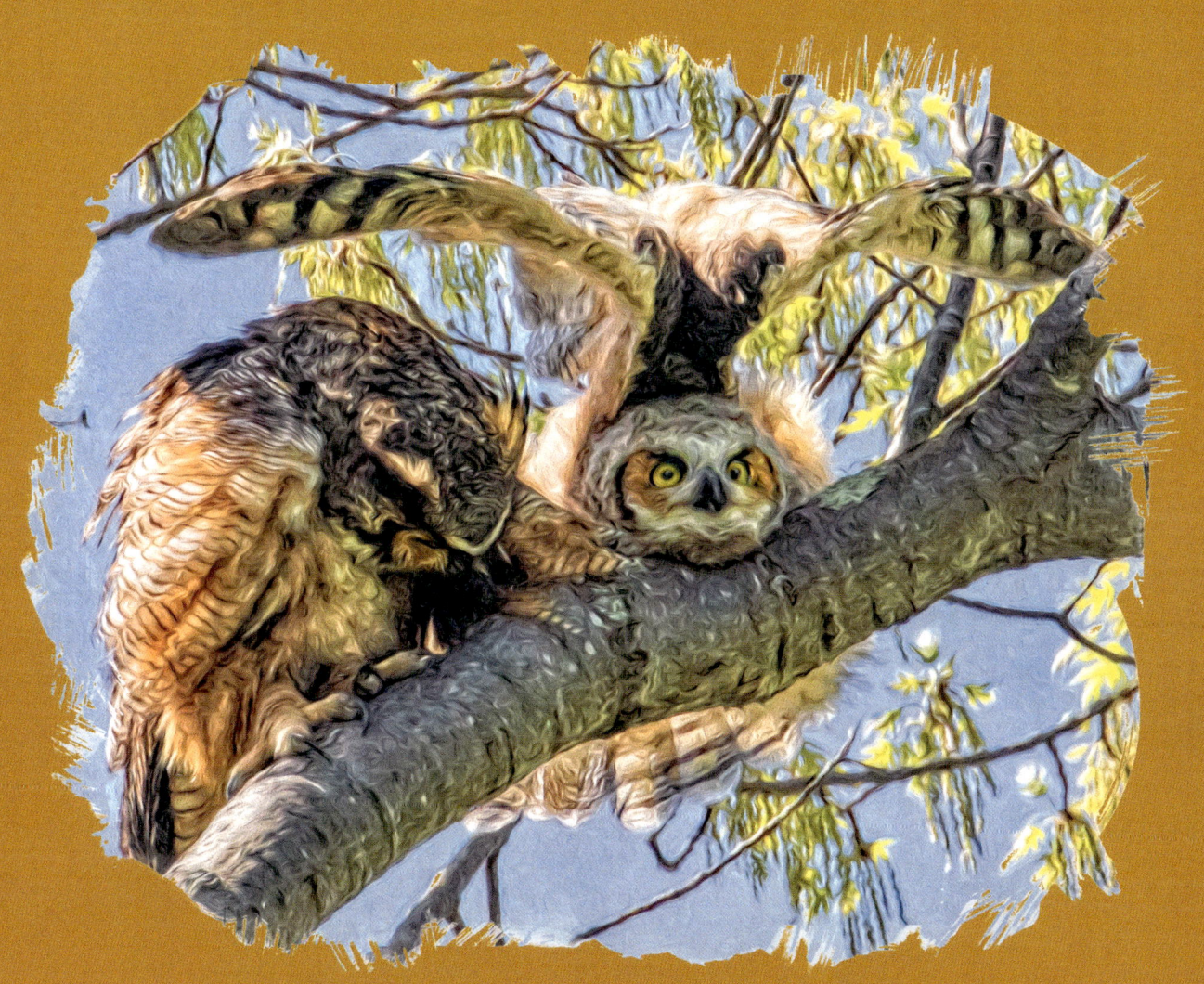

The owl's human friends were so happy for Skylar, even though they didn't see the owlet as often. Owlets needed to stay quiet to stay safe. Spring continued, the trees leafed out completely, and Skylar began the Great Adventure of Life.

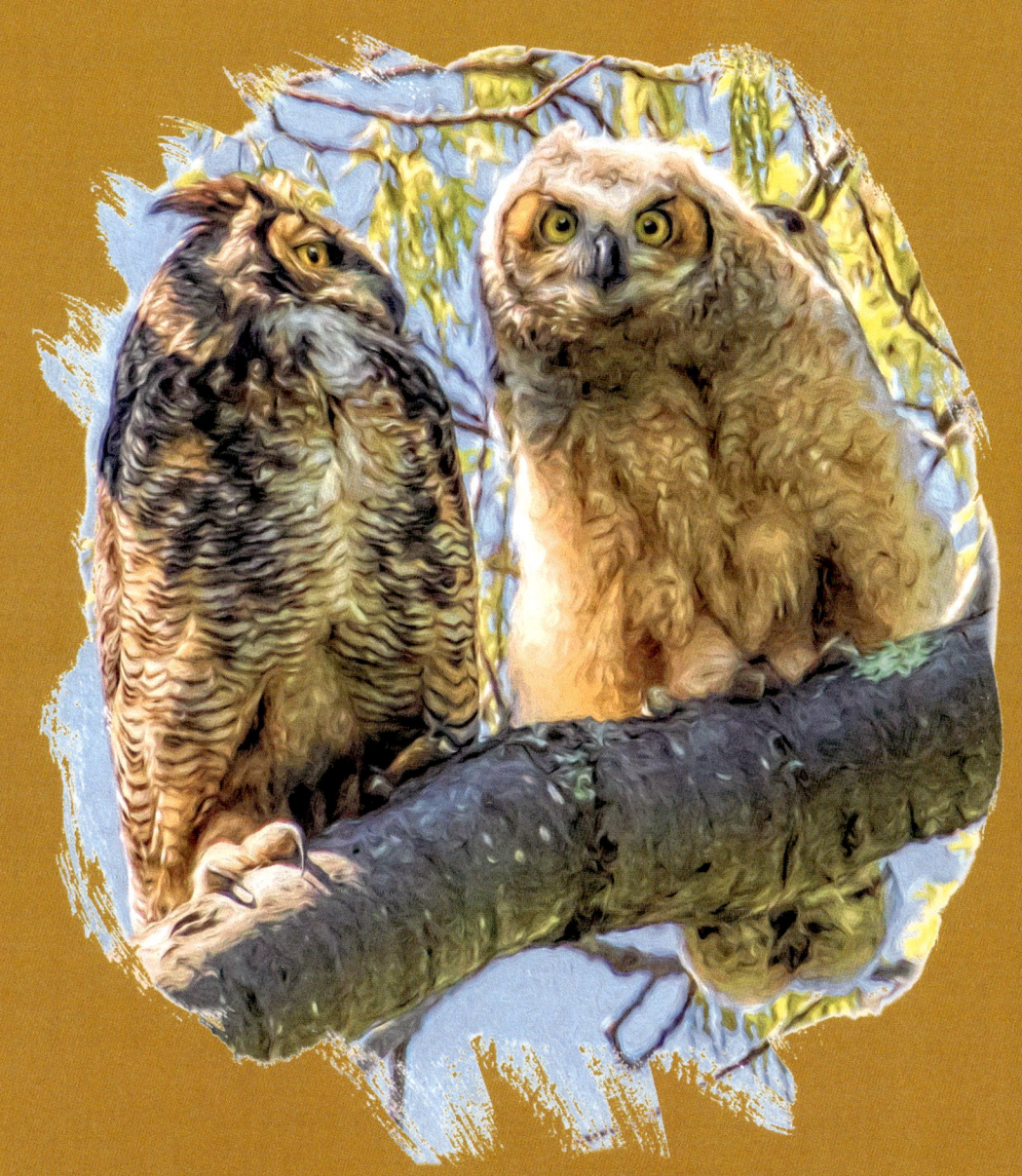

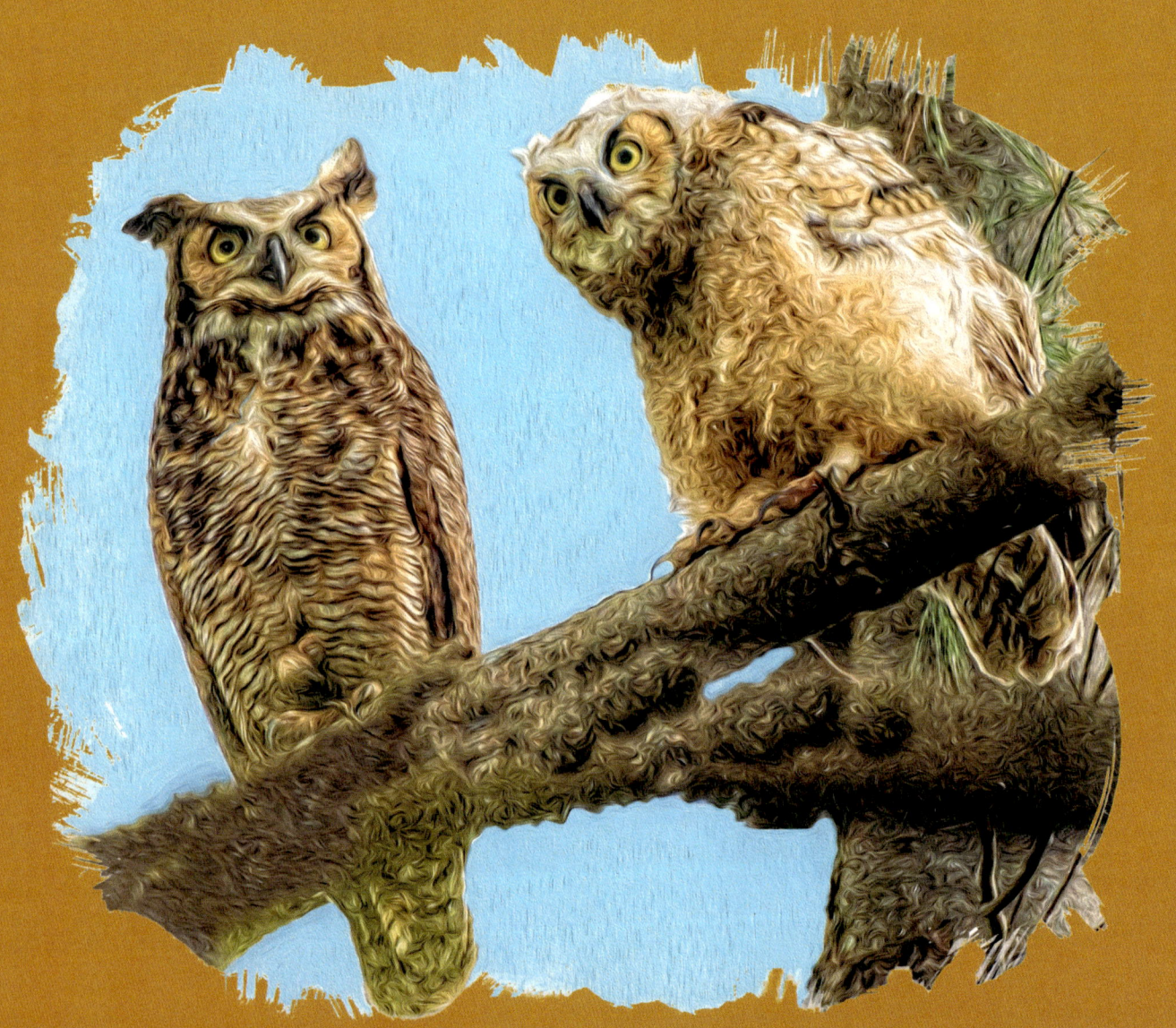

OWL FACTS

- The Great Horned Owl is the most common of North American owls.

- Great Horned Owls do not have actual "horns;" they are actually tufted feathers.

- Great Horned Owls are nocturnal, which means they are active at night.

- Great Horned Owl pairs stay together, and they make excellent parents.

- Great Horned Owls eat a variety of prey, including rodents, small mammals, & even geese and skunks!

- Great Horned Owls swallow their prey whole, and later regurgitate (cough-up) "pellets" that are composed of fur, bones, and other unused parts of their meal.

- Great Horned Owls are threatened by habitat loss, and by eating rodents that had been poisoned by rodenticide.

- You can help owls, other birds, yourselves and the environment by eating fruits and vegetables that have not been sprayed with pesticides and herbicides.

ACKNOWLEDGMENTS

The authors would like to thank the following individuals who contributed to this project:

Vinnie Falcione, Fresh Pond Reservation Site Supervisor for the Cambridge Water Department; Chief Ranger Jean Rogers; and Ranger/ Outreach & Volunteer Coordinator Tim Puopolo, for helping to protect the grounded owlet before it could learn to fly.

A special shout-out to Ranger Tim Puopolo for his informative presentation, The Owlet Debriefed, on June 30, 2018.

Grateful thanks to Joan Fleiss Kaplan and Wendy Drexler, authors of **Buzz, Ruby and Their City Chicks**, for their advice and counsel.

We also thank Amy Saltzman, Editor of the Cambridge Chronicle, who knew that Skylar's story was a great human story; a great wildlife story; and a great Cambridge story.

Thank you, Susan Moses, for contributing comprehensive notes about Skylar and the timeline of events.

Special thanks to our first readers: Cathy Minogue; Kirsten Cecchin; Bobbie Gatz, and Lily Veronica Prisco. We appreciate your valuable feedback.

Our gratitude for: Corinne and Artty Kinsman, Peter Filichia, Linda Konner, Bob and Edie Di Giorgio, James Harrison, Mary Hogan, Joe Plati, Joe and Karen Polvere, Keith and Cathy Joyce, Bob, Becky and Virginia Parsons, Mark Nickerson, Don and Geri Tremblay, Paul Roberts, Wayne Petersen, Craig Gibson, Ellen Blackstone of Birdnote, Ray Brown of Talkin' Birds, Howie Carr, William Martin, Upton Bell, Gary Goshgarian, Lloyd and Joyce Torgove, Frank and Bobbie Gatz, Sharon Sherman, John Amaral and - always - Steve Gladstone, who brings ideas and manuscripts to life.

Thank you, Michael Armanious and Arlington Community Media Inc., for your enthusiastic support and for making our Dead in Good Company video.

A shout-out to our dedicated contributing photographers who are in the field day by day searching for the wonders of wildlife. John Harrison: Cover photo and the photos on pages 7, 9. 23, 25, 27, 29, 31, 33, 37, 39, 41, 45, 49, 51, 53, 59, 61, 63., 65; Kim Nagy: Back cover photo and the photos on pages 43, 55, 57; Sandy Selesky: 67, 69; Andy Provost: 19, 21, 70; Jim Renault: 13; Eric Olick: 35; Ken Stampfer: 5; Mark Resendes: 15; and Susan Moses: 11,17,47.

And lastly, to the memory of our wonderful friend Ernie Sarro.

ABOUT THE AUTHORS

John Harrison and Kim Nagy are the Editors of **Dead in Good Company**, a compelling collection of essays, poems and wildlife photographs of Mount Auburn Cemetery in Cambridge, Massachusetts. Sweet Auburn, as it's affectionately known, is America's first garden cemetery, and **Dead in Good Company** is the first book to celebrate the Cemetery as a place of regeneration and transformation; the circle of life. Mount Auburn Cemetery is one of New England's Birding Hotspots.

See more at: www.facebook.com/deadingoodcompany and on YouTube: https://www.youtube.com/watch?v=cFwi69Uk2-4&feature=youtu.be&app=desktop

John Harrison Founded Epilog Enterprises, a book distribution company, in 1975. His passion for nature ultimately led to the idea for **Dead in Good Company**. His photographs have been published by Mass Audubon, the Humane Society of the United States, and Project Coyote in CA, and have appeared in books, calendars, magazines, newspapers, and websites. He lectures on nature and wildlife at elementary schools and to senior citizen groups. Additionally, he initiated and has authored the *Medford Wildlife Watch* blog for *The Medford Transcript* newspaper since 2009.

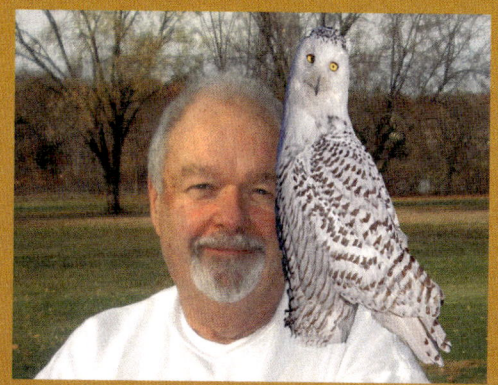

Kim Nagy has made the natural world both her profession and her hobby. She is an avid wildlife and nature photographer, and travels widely in pursuit of her craft. She works as a regional sales manager in the natural foods industry, covering the East Coast & Midwest. Her photos have appeared in National Geographic's *Daily Dozen*, *BirdWatching*, *The BirdNote* calendar, several publications of the Massachusetts Audubon Society, *The Marco Review*, and more.

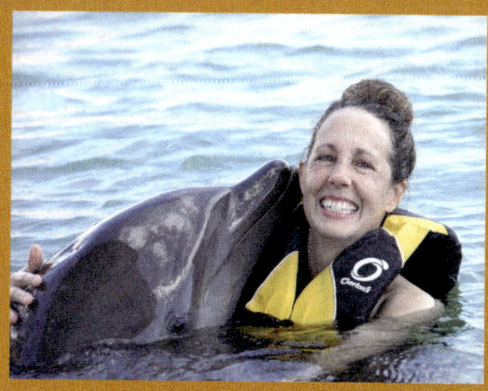

See more at: www.facebook.com/catchlightphotos

73

48438343R00042

Made in the USA
Middletown, DE
15 June 2019